# www.harcourt- 

Bringing you products from all Harcourt Health Sciences
companies including Baillière Tindall, Churchill Livingstone,
Mosby and W.B. Saunders

- ● **Browse** for latest information on new books, journals
  and electronic products

- ● **Search** for information on over 20 000 published
  titles with full product information including tables
  of contents and sample chapters

- ● **Keep up to date** with our extensive publishing
  programme in your field by registering with eAlert
  or requesting postal updates

- ● **Secure online ordering** with prompt delivery, as well
  as full contact details to order by phone, fax or post

- ● **News** of special features and promotions

If you are based in the following countries, please visit the
country-specific site to receive full details of product
availability and local ordering information

USA: www.harcourthealth.com

Canada: www.harcourtcanada.com

Australia: www.harcourt.com.au

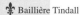 Baillière Tindall  CHURCHILL LIVINGSTONE  Mosby 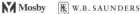 W.B. SAUNDERS

# Churchill Livingstone's A–Z Guide to Professional Healthcare

Editor

## Maggy Wallace MA BA RN DipN RCNT DipED RNT
Professional development adviser

Foreword by

## Pippa Gough MSc PGCEA RN RM HV
Fellow, King's Fund

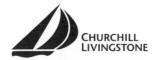
**CHURCHILL LIVINGSTONE**

EDINBURGH LONDON NEW YORK PHILADELPHIA ST LOUIS SYDNEY TORONTO 2002

CHURCHILL LIVINGSTONE
An imprint of Harcourt Publishers Limited

 is a registered trademark of Harcourt Publishers
Limited

ISBN 0 443 06402 4

**British Library Cataloguing in Publication Data**
A catalogue record for this book is available from
the British Library

**Library of Congress Cataloging in Publication Data**
A catalog record for this book is available from
the Library of Congress

The
publisher's
policy is to use
**paper manufactured
from sustainable forests**

Printed in China
by RDC Group Limited

# Foreword

Over the last decade we have become familiar with the concept of the 'one-stop shop' in relation to clinical care and services. It is the epitome of 'modern' care embracing as it does ideas of expertness, accessibility, flexibility, user-friendliness and responsiveness. This amazing book is the literary equivalent – the one-stop shop of useful information for busy healthcare practitioners and many others from related fields.

The scope of the book is truly mind-blowing. Some subjects must have been omitted from the final compilation but it is hard to fathom out what these could have been. I couldn't come up with anything! As such, it will be an endless source of good quality information for many people who do not have the time to search through numerous books and publications to find the answers to their questions.

I worked with Maggy Wallace for a number of years at the United Kingdom Central Council for Nursing, Midwifery and Health Visiting (see page 151). She was always the one I turned to for the information I needed. She has an eclectic knowledge which is staggering in its breadth and scope. It is so heart-warming to see that Maggy has converted this into something which is now available to others – it makes me feel less selfish, less indulged, somehow. Thank you Maggy, for this invaluable, idiosyncratic and fascinating resource. Only you could have conceived of it, stuck with it (when any lesser mortal would have peered into the abyss and slunk away) and delivered it with such aplomb and brilliance.

PG, 2002

# Preface

Healthcare is changing so rapidly, both in terms of the organisation and delivery of care and the knowledge base needed by healthcare professionals, that keeping up to date is a real and significant challenge.

Access to clear, understandable, accurate information in a concise and readable format is essential. This is particularly so for those coming new to the field as students, those qualified/registered individuals who are returning to practice, and for those who are trying to keep up to date with the changes. Information is available but it is scattered throughout a number of disparate sources, all of which take time and effort to access – and time is the main commodity which is in short supply in the lives of busy healthcare professionals.

*The main purpose of this Guide, therefore, is to provide a single source of user-friendly information on issues of significance to healthcare professionals.*

It is deliberately designed to be multiprofessional in nature and address those issues which are relevant to all healthcare professionals, with the exception of clinical issues, which are dealt with in detail in numerous other sources. The increasing emphasis on partnership, team working and seamless care fortunately makes professional tribalism increasingly a thing of the past. This book will, we hope, contribute to that significant and welcome shift in both attitude and organisation.

One of the challenges of a book of this nature is what to include and what to omit, and to an extent there is no limit on what could be included. In the end, however, pragmatic decisions have to be made or it would still be in the process of being written! Hopefully there is enough here to keep you, the reader, well informed and hungry for more – the essence of lifelong learning!

MW, 2002

# Introduction

Welcome to this unusual and, we think, distinctive book. Designed as a reference book for all those interested in the effective delivery of good quality healthcare, it will appeal to all healthcare professionals – both those studying to enter a profession and those qualified and/or registered practitioners wanting to up-date their knowledge. It is both informative and user friendly and we are confident that it will prove an invaluable resource, finding a welcome home with many healthcare professionals.

It is not the intention to give exhaustive detail on each issue – there are numerous other books on the market designed to do just that. It is designed to give you just enough information to know the essence of a particular issue, so that you can decide whether you need to look further. Neither is it designed to address clinical issues – again there is a plethora of other sources available.

It is idiosyncratic in its style in that contributions have come from a number and range of experts before editing. It is also deliberately idiosyncratic in the treatment, approach and length of each contribution – complex subjects such as ethics and health, for example, get more space and attention than factual information. We believe that this adds to the richness of the book as a source of information. There is a distinct bias towards issues which can be broadly considered under the heading of 'professional development' – reflecting the editor's own passionate belief in the importance of such matters, particularly in the rapidly changing context within which we all work. There is also an emphasis on the involvement of consumers/users in the health partnership – another of the editor's interests!

The topics are arranged in A–Z order for ease of reference, with cross referencing where necessary.

## Icons

The following icons are used in the A–Z guide:

▨     indicates that the entry is a charity or organisation.

✉     indicates that the postal address for the organisation is listed in Appendix 1.

☎     indicates that the telephone number for the organisation is listed in Appendix 1.

▤     indicates that the fax number for the organisation is listed in Appendix 1.

@     indicates that the e-mail address for the organisation is listed in Appendix 1.

🖱     indicates that the website address for the organisation is listed in Appendix 1.

# Acknowledgements

This book could not have been written without the generous and knowledgeable help and interest of many friends and colleagues. To you all, thank you. In terms of contributions, the generosity of friends came as no surprise but was no less appreciated. The generosity of those whom I have never met, yet who offered to contribute when hearing of the project, came as a pleasant and quite unexpected bonus. To you all, an even bigger thank you.

As always, thanks to Jacqueline Curthoys, my editor, ever patient and positive.

And finally, but importantly, thanks to my family and friends who support me on a regular basis with their continued interest in my work and who suffer with me when deadlines loom and the going is difficult.

MW, 2002

# Contributors

Ingrid Anstey
Alison Askew
Gill Collinson
Mark Darley
Tina Funnell
Bernice Grant
Susan Hamer
Cathy Hull
Julie Hyde
Carol Kirby
Jeanette Laird-Measures
Catherine McLoughlin
Elaine McNichol
Chris Marsh

Ann Matthews
Christina Milne
Hannah Miskin
Chris Morris
Anne Rabbetts
Lesley Radley
Liz Redfern
Trevor Ride
Lynn Rowley
Oliver Slevin
Graham Smith
Sue Smith
Marina Williams
Tim Young

# A–Z guide contents

## Access to Health Records Act 1990

The Access to Health Records Act gives patients and clients the right of access to manual health records about themselves which were made after 1 November 1991. The system for dealing with applications is set out in the *Access to Health Records Act 1990: a Guide for the NHS* published by the government health department (DOH 1990). All healthcare practitioners must be aware of, and honour, the rights of patients and clients on this issue.

## Accountability

Individual professionals are accountable for their own professional practice. They are expected to be able to account for their actions to any enquirer and to justify them on the grounds of best practice and knowledge, informed by good clinical judgement. In addition, each individual has an accountability to their professional peers, their team or department, the organisation which employs them and their statutory body and/or their professional organisation. There is also a wider accountability to the individual and organisational users of the service, potential users, taxpayers, the government and society as a whole. (See Clinical governance and Clinical supervision.)

These can alternatively be classified as accountability to:

- the public, through criminal law, e.g. murder
- the patient, through civil law, e.g. negligence, breaching the duty of care
- the employer, through contractual law, e.g. breaching confidentiality
- the profession, through professional 'law', e.g. inappropriate treatment of a patient.

These accountabilities are not necessarily mutually exclusive and a single event may require practitioners to answer for their actions in a number of ways. The codes of conduct or ethics (see entries) used by individual professions are based upon the concept of accountability.

## ▨ Action for Victims of Medical Accidents

Action for Victims of Medical Accidents (AVMA) is a charity specialising in providing independent advice and support to patients injured during the course of medical treatment. AVMA maintains a database of over 2500 medico-legal experts, and has a library of medical and legal textbooks supplemented by medical journals, law reports, government publications, Medline and the Internet. ✉ ☾ 📄 @ ✍

## Advance Directives ('Living Will')

Informed consent is the basis of all medical treatment for mentally competent adults. Patients can make it clear what treatment they wish or do not wish to have in the event of a change in their health status – and this can be written as an Advance Directive, or Living Will. Advance Directives have a basis in common law but this may be of little help to patients unable, because of their condition, to fight a case through the courts. The matter is still currently being discussed following the Law Commission's recommended legislation in 1995.

## Advocacy

An advocate, in a generic rather than a specifically legal sense, is one who supports or champions another, often because an individual, for whatever reason, is not in a position to speak adequately or effectively for him or herself. Advocacy in healthcare is about promoting and protecting the interests of patients and clients who may be both vulnerable and incapable of effectively protecting their own interests – either because of their physical or mental health state or because they have no friends or family to support them. Advocacy is not a role confined to a particular healthcare profession and can take a number of forms. It may mean ensuring that the patient or client has adequate information upon which to make knowledgeable, informed decisions about his or her own healthcare. It may mean supporting an individual who has decided not to accept the treatment or care offered. It will mean respecting the decision that an autonomous

A

individual makes about his/her own healthcare, providing that the individual has had access to all the relevant information and is in a position to make an informed choice. This can vary according to the patient/client's age and health state. (See Patient Advocacy and Liaison Service.)

## Ambulance services

Ambulance services are required for the transportation of emergency and urgent cases to hospital, and for inter-hospital transportation. They are also required for a large number of non-emergency cases, e.g. non-ambulant patients being discharged, or being transported to and from outpatient and day hospital attendances. There are around 37 ambulance services in England, 5 in Wales, 1 in Northern Ireland and 1 in Scotland. By 1997 all of these had become NHS Trusts or had become part of a larger Trust.

Non-emergency journeys make up around 80% of all journeys.

Concerns about the ambulance services have in the past focused on the following:

- status of an emergency service
- operational cost-effectiveness
- response times.

The Patient's Charter requires that, in 95% of cases, emergency ambulances should reach patients within 14 minutes in urban areas and 19 in rural areas.

The ambulance services have undergone considerable changes in the 1980s and early 1990s. A variety of measures have been introduced to improve efficiency:

- Ambulance controls are fully automated.
- Emergency ambulance vehicles are equipped and manned by specially trained crews with paramedical skills.
- Volunteer drivers and vehicles are used for non-urgent 'hospital transport'.
- A variety of vehicles, e.g. helicopters, high speed cars and motorcycles, are used to improve response time.

Emphasis is on stabilising the patient on arrival and preparing for transportation to the appropriate service. The ambulance service is required to respond to all 999 calls made by members of the public. Calls are logged automatically. It is expected that all ambulance controls will be able to prioritise 999 calls.

## APL, APEL

APL and APEL – often written as AP(E)L – refer to the Assessment of Prior (Experiential) Learning. The learning can either have been certificated in some way (APL) or can be from experience (hence experiential) (APEL). An individual, therefore, who wants to achieve a particular qualification can ask to have previous relevant learning taken into account or credited – perhaps from a course or courses he or she may have undertaken previously, or from relevant work or life experience. Clearly the learning has to be demonstrable and this can be done in a number of ways – through the use of portfolios of learning, the writing of assignments or the presentation of case studies, for example. AP(E)L processes are time consuming for those involved and because they are resource intensive can be expensive, although the actual cost varies considerably from institution to institution. (See also CATS.)

### Association of Healthcare Human Resource Management

Formed in the mid-1970s, the Association of Healthcare Human Resource Management (AHHRM) is an organisation designed to bring together healthcare professionals to enable them to develop, influence and promote high quality human resource management within the NHS. The body is a major player in health service management and has strategic alliances with a number of other leading management associations and trade unions. It is consulted on all important national human resource (HR) issues. ✉ ☞

### Association of Medical Research Charities

The Association of Medical Research Charities (AMRC) was founded in 1972 and established as a formal organisation in 1987. It aims to further medical research in the UK generally and in particular to advance the effectiveness of those charities for whom medical research is a principal activity. The AMRC aims to represent members collectively in the fora responsible for the formulation of national policy and the direction of UK medical research. It has 105 members and provides a collective voice for their contribution and a single point of contact for those needing to consult the charitable sector on medical research. ✉ ☽ 📄 @

## Audit

Audit is the process of comparing existing practice with an agreed standard. As an organisation which has accountability for public funds, the business and financial practices of NHS organisations are subject to audit. However, when audit is mentioned in relation to healthcare it is usually referring to clinical audit. The National Centre for Clinical Audit offers this definition of *clinical audit*: 'A clinically led initiative which seeks to improve the quality and outcome of patient care through structured peer review whereby clinicians examine their practices and results against explicit standards and modify their practice where indicated'.

Clinical audit evolved from medical audit which entailed physicians examining their practice aside from other professionals. It soon became apparent that good patient care resulted from integrated practice from many professionals and the emphasis shifted to clinical audit. Typically, audits are conducted to evaluate the effectiveness of medicines or treatments. However, almost any aspect of clinical care can be audited. Discharge planning, patient teaching, wound care, nutrition and pain management are other examples of clinical audit topics.

The fundamental first step in effective clinical audit is to identify and agree a standard. This is often the most valuable part of the process because it requires clinicians of all relevant professions to discuss and compare practices, which in itself can improve the consistency and quality of care. The key stages in the audit process are:

- deciding on a topic to audit, the reasons for doing the audit, how the care will be measured and which cases should be included
- collecting data on practice, often from medical records or observing care
- evaluating the findings against the standard and identifying causes of incompatible performance

- acting to improve care
- repeating the data collection, evaluation and action steps as often as needed to consistently raise the standard.

Where organisations often fall short is in the action stage. It can be challenging and time consuming to change clinical practice. Experienced professionals become confident with practice patterns that have given them good results in the past. When faced with the prospect of change, there is often a need for education, persuasion and support to make it happen.

The importance of clinical audit as a tool for improving patient care has re-emerged with the introduction of clinical governance (see entry). The setting of clinical standards and the evaluation of practice against those standards is a fundamental activity which is necessary to meet the expectations within clinical governance. The most important role of clinical audit is, however, to assure the best standards of care through a systematic, interactive, peer supported process.

## Audit Commission

The Audit Commission appoints auditors to all local authorities and NHS bodies in England and Wales and helps bring about improvements in economy, efficiency and effectiveness through value for money studies and the audit process. ✉ 🖱

# A–Z guide

## ▨ Baby Network

The Baby Network is a loose alliance of all the voluntary organisations working on issues affecting babies and pregnancy. ✉ ☾ 🖹 @

## ▨ BackCare

BackCare (until recently known as National Backpain Association) helps people manage and prevent back pain. It does this by providing advice, promoting self help, encouraging debate and funding scientific research into better back care. @ ☜

## ▨ Beacons

This is the name given to NHS organisations in England, which may be Trusts or GP practices, who are considered, after a rigorous selection process, to be examples of good practice. Evidence has to be produced which demonstrates:

- that patients are receiving a better than average service
- that the scheme is replicable, and
- that the individuals concerned are eager to share their good practice.

## Benchmarking

A benchmark is a standard or point of reference used as a means of testing. Benchmarking is used to describe a process whereby organisations identify best performers or best practice in order to improve quality. The way that results are achieved are subject to scrutiny in order that others can bring their own performance in line with the best.

## ▨ Blood Transfusion Service

The National Blood Transfusion Service began in 1946. Currently the service in England is managed by the National Blood

**B**

Authority (NBA), which was created in 1993 to replace the Central Blood Laboratories Authority and the National Directorate of the National Blood Transfusion Service.

The NBA has become responsible for 15 Regional Transfusion Centres (RTCs) since 1994. The objectives of the NBA are to:

- maintain and promote blood and blood product supply based on a system of voluntary donors
- implement a cost-effective national strategy to ensure adequate supply
- meet national needs
- ensure high standards of safety and quality
- ensure cost-efficient operation of the Blood Centres, the Bio-Products Laboratory and the International Blood Group Reference Laboratory as parts of the national service.

Under plans approved in 1995 to reorganise the blood service, there are now three geographical zones with administration centres in Bristol, Leeds and Colindale (North London). Bulk processing and testing has been consolidated in 10 centres but the 15 RTCs retain various functions in addition to storing and supplying functions. A national computer system has been introduced to improve organisation of donation, inventory and stock control.

The NHS uses around 5000 litres of blood a day and demand has been rising by around 4% each year. Only 5% of the population are donors, hence the NBA's struggle is constantly to recruit and retain more donors. Blood also has a relatively short shelf life, and also needs to be compatible with the recipient's own blood group.

The Blood Centres are reimbursed by the hospitals for the products ordered and used.

## British Association for Counselling

The British Association for Counselling (BAC) aims to promote education and training for those involved in counselling, full- or part-time, in either professional or voluntary contexts, with a view to raising standards. A further aim is to promote the understanding of counselling.

It organises conferences and specialist events to provide informed comment on many current issues. Members have experience of a wide range of counselling practice in settings such as unemployment, alcoholism, drug abuse, relationships, bereavement, AIDS/HIV, counselling in the health service and in education settings. ✉ ☏ 📄 @ ☝

## British Association of Occupational Therapists/College of Occupational Therapists

The College of Occupational Therapists, a subsidiary of the British Association of Occupational Therapists, is concerned with the professional practice and education of occupational therapists. It sets standards of practice for the profession; promotes the profession as a career; supports educational and research activities from undergraduate to postgraduate level; works with other statutory and professional bodies; represents the profession at government level, as well as providing advice to members on professional and ethical matters.

The College, in partnership with the Council for Professions Supplementary to Medicine and with educational establishments, is responsible for the validation and monitoring of all pre-registration degrees in occupational therapy.

The organisation publishes a monthly academic journal, the *British Journal of Occupational Therapy* and a monthly house magazine *Occupational Therapy News* for its 20 000 recipients, who include occupational therapists, their support workers and student registrants. ✉ ☏ 📄 ☝

## British Dental Association

The British Dental Association (BDA) is the trades union and professional association which represents the interests of dentists throughout the UK. Members work in general dental practice, in the community dental service, in universities, hospitals, the armed forces and industry. It provides scientific and professional advice for dentists and can also provide briefings for Members of Parliament for parliamentary debates and parliamentary questions if required. ☏ ☝

## British Dietetic Association

The British Dietetic Association (BDA) is both the professional association representing State Registered Dietitians and an independent trade union. The Association was formed in 1936 and has grown steadily to the point where they have over 4000 members, of whom about 65% work in the NHS. As with other professional associations, the BDA offers a wide range of services to its members ranging from individual terms such as professional indemnity insurance through to broader strategic matters like representing the profession's interests to the Government. ✉ ☽ 🖹 🖑

## British Heart Foundation

The British Heart Foundation finances and encourages research into the causes, prevention, diagnosis and treatment of cardiovascular disease. It disseminates knowledge about the prevention and treatment of heart disease to the public. ✉ ☽ 🖹 🖑

## British Lung Foundation

The British Lung Foundation exists to fund research into all lung diseases. It provides public information on lung diseases and good lung health and it supports people with a lung condition through the Breathe Easy Club. ✉ ☽ 🖹 @ 🖑

## British Medical Association

The British Medical Association (BMA) is a voluntary professional association for doctors which aims to promote the science of medicine and to maintain the honour and interests of the medical profession. ✉ ☽ 🖑

## British Nutrition Foundation

The British Nutrition Foundation promotes the nutritional well-being of society through the impartial interpretation and effective dissemination of scientifically based nutritional knowledge and advice. It works in partnership with academic and research institutes, the food industry, educators and government. The Foundation influences all in the food chain, government, the professions and the media. The Foundation is a charitable organisation, which receives funds from the food industry, government and a variety of other sources. ✉ ☽ 🖹 @

##  British Psychological Society

The British Psychological Society (BPS) was founded in 1901 and incorporated by Royal Charter in 1965. It exists to:

B

- promote the advancement and dissemination of psychology and its applications
- maintain high standards of professional education and conduct
- maintain a register of Chartered Psychologists under amendments to its Royal Charter in 1987.

✉ ☽ 🗒

# A-Z guide

## ▨ CancerBACUP

CancerBACUP specialises in high quality information and support for people affected by cancer. It provides a national free-phone helpline staffed by specialist cancer nurses, and has a wide range and number of booklets and fact sheets on types of cancer, treatments and living with the disease. ✉ ☽ 📄 @ ⬦

## ▨ Cancerlink

Cancerlink's mission is to strengthen the network of support based on shared experience of cancer, to help anyone affected by cancer to access that support and to use their unique experience to help shape future cancer services. ✉ ☽ 📄 @ ⬦

## Capital

Capital is the term given to money which is spent in order to acquire items that:

- have a life of more than 1 year such as land/premises and large pieces of equipment
- cost (either individually or as a group) more than a specified amount.

Capital money is spent also in order to carry out work on premises, such as adaptation, renewal, replacement and demolition.

In the NHS there are stringent rules which must be adhered to when spending capital. There are levels of spending laid down which 'trigger' certain processes. Items or services which will cost more than a certain amount will require certain procedures to be carried out. For example, all big building contracts are required now to be advertised in relevant European journals, and full tendering processes must be invoked. Smaller projects such as the purchase of small amounts of furniture may only require that three quotes/estimates are obtained, providing that the supplier is on the NHS suppliers' list. The amounts are reviewed regularly to take inflation into account. (See also Revenue.)

## ▨ Carers National Association

The Carers National Association is the voice of carers and is the leading national charity of and for people who look after relatives and friends with disabilities or long-term illness or who are elderly and frail. They provide information and advice to carers by letter and on a telephone advice line – mainly about welfare rights. There is a CNA members' magazine – *Caring* (see Appendix 1). ⊠ ☾ @ ✐

## CATS and APEL see Credit Accumulation and Transfer Schemes

## Chaplaincy

At its simplest level the role of the hospital chaplaincy service is to provide for the spiritual needs of patients, staff and relatives/friends and to be available and accessible 24 hours a day, every day. The Hospital Chaplain is a priest to the entire institution and to all who work in it, at all levels, offering support and impartial confidentiality for those who wish to share personal or professional struggles with someone who is outside their management structure.

Sometimes spiritual needs will be met in an overtly religious fashion, such as offering the sacraments, praying with individuals and anointing the dying. Often, however, they will be addressed in less obvious ways, enabling people to wrestle with the existential issues relating to life, purpose and meaning, sickness and death. Hospital Chaplains liaise with local clergy and leaders of other faiths at the requests of patients and relatives whilst at all times maintaining patient confidentiality. Chaplains are not there to evangelise, to impose truth or interpretation, but rather to accompany others in their search for meaning.

The Chaplain will have counselling and communications skills, be able to break bad news and remain in situations of pain and despair where words are inadequate and clichés offensive. The Chaplain is a symbol of human spiritual aspiration who shares in the depths as well as the heights of human experience.

## ▨ Chartered Society of Physiotherapy

The Chartered Society of Physiotherapy was established in 1894. Its aim is to support and promote members and their profession to ensure the best possible care is available to patients wherever they are. ✉ ➀ 📄 ⟨⟩

## Clinical governance

The NHS English White Paper, *The New NHS: Modern, Dependable* (DOH 1997) made a strong point of putting quality at the heart of organisational practice. Like many new initiatives before it, is analogous to corporate governance in the business world. Clinical governance is an initiative to assure and improve clinical standards at local level throughout the NHS. It has been conceived as an umbrella term to describe a range of activities including audit, clinical effectiveness, clinical guidelines and protocols and clinical risk management. It includes action to ensure that systems are in place to ensure continuous improvements in clinical care; that risks are avoided; that adverse events are rapidly detected, openly investigated and lessons learned; and that good practice is rapidly disseminated.

The 1998 and ongoing high profile General Medical Council debate about cardiac consultants' operative procedures on babies in Bristol raised the issue of clinical and managerial accountability of consultants to their patients and families. It raised the responsibility of managers to see that clinical audit was happening effectively, an area of work that had previously remained firmly in the clinicians' domain. Following Bristol and publication of the White Paper on clinical governance the statutory duty for quality of care is now something that Chief Executives and Trust Boards need to take very seriously. The Chief Executive is held legally accountable for ensuring effective systems are in place. In many places a sub-committee of the Board, made up of executive and non-executive directors, is set up to deal with the clinical governance/effectiveness/quality agenda.

However, quality in healthcare is a relatively contemporary concept. The Griffiths Report (DOH 1983) not only introduced general management to the NHS but also increased the drive towards quality assurance. Since then many organisations have developed packages to help clinical and managerial staff identify the quality standards of care for client groups and have assisted in, for example, the King's Fund Organisational Audit or Health Services Accreditation.

There is significant challenge for health boards to support staff in this clinical work, to provide education and time to carry out clinical audit, to promote and disseminate evidence based practice and to oversee and authorise internal clinical guidelines and policies.

## Clinical guidelines see Protocols

## Clinical pathways see Protocols

## Clinical and performance indicators

Clinical and performance indicators are designed to monitor and improve standards of care for NHS patients. They provide figures at NHS Trust level, rather than individual clinician or clinician team level.

The clinical indicators concentrate on six key areas:

- deaths in hospital following surgery
- deaths in hospital following a fractured hip
- deaths in hospital following a heart attack
- readmission to hospital
- returning home following treatment for a stroke
- returning home following treatment for a broken hip.

The performance indicators look at a wider range of activities, grouped under six main headings:

- health improvement, including: registrations of cancer, deaths from circulatory diseases and accidents; and suicide
- fair access, including: surgery rates, waiting lists, adults and children registered with an NHS dentist, and early detection of cancer
- effective delivery of appropriate care, including: cost-effective prescribing, discharge from hospital, and levels of inappropriate surgery
- efficiency, including: length of stay in hospital, unit costs of maternity and specialist mental health services, and generic prescribing

- patient/care experience, including: patients who wait for more than 2 hours in A&E for admission, operations cancelled for non-medical reasons, delayed discharges, and numbers of patients on waiting lists of 12 months or more
- health outcomes of NHS care, including: avoidable deaths, conceptions below age 16, adverse events/complications, and infant deaths.

## ▧ Clinical Standards Board for Scotland

The Clinical Standards Board for Scotland was established in April 1999 as a special health board. Its role is to develop standards and maintain clinical standards across Scotland, to support staff in their efforts to improve quality, and to reassure the public that services are being delivered safely and to the highest standards. The Board is made up of 50% NHS staff and 50% from outside. Early work has concentrated on developing a template for standard setting and peer review. Pilot reviews have also been commissioned on coronary heart disease and mental health. ✉ ◑ 🗎 @

## Clinical supervision

Most of the healthcare professions have some means of supporting practitioners and students in clinical practice, although the level of support varies from profession to profession. Good clinical supervision should be separated from the managerial role and is designed to support all practising professionals, offering a safe and supportive environment in which issues relating to their practice can be discussed.

Clinical supervision works well when the two participants have negotiated a shared and explicit understanding of the purpose of the activity, and have clear boundaries and specific review points. In this way, arrangements can be made which meet the unique needs of the individuals concerned within certain agreed parameters.

Ideally, specific preparation should be given to those undertaking the supervisory role, whether supporting students or supporting registered/qualified practitioners. The literature identifies a range of desirable skills and personal attributes for those effectively undertaking the supervisory role. They include: a sense of humour, patience, open mindedness, approachability, self-awareness, honesty, objectivity, maturity, sincerity, warmth, trustworthiness and understanding. Individuals need to be professional, non-threatening and non-judgemental, flexible, self-confident, committed, assertive and prepared to give regular feedback. In addition, supervisors need to be good role models commanding peer respect, have demonstrable clinical competence, show good interpersonal skills, be facilitators of learning and the development of initiative and independence and be reflective practitioners (NBS 1999).

## Cochrane database

This is a database of systematic reviews of published research provided by an international multidisciplinary collaboration of health professionals, consumers and researchers who review randomised controlled clinical trials.

## Codes of conduct

Having a code of conduct or ethics is one of the key criteria for an occupational group to consider itself a profession. Such codes are used as the basis for describing a template of the expectations placed upon, and behaviour required of, individual members of the profession. They set out in varying degrees of detail what is expected of practitioners within that particular profession and are frequently used as the basis against which allegations of professional misconduct or incompetence are judged. They emphasise the accountability of the individuals and the behaviour which can be expected from each member of that profession. Breaches of a profession's code of conduct/ethics can result in disciplinary action, ranging from local disciplinary measures, such as formal warnings or even dismissal, through to being reported to the relevant statutory body, such as the General Dental Council, the United Kingdom Central Council for Nursing, Midwifery and Health Visiting or the General Medical Council, with the possibility of removal from the professional register of the profession concerned and the consequential loss of the right to practise.

## College of Health

The College of Health is a charity with the aims of:

- relieving sickness
- protecting people's health

- undertaking the advancement of health education
- preventing illness
- assisting in the care of the sick, handicapped and disabled.

## ⊠ Commission for Health Improvement

The Commission for Health Improvement (CHI) is a statutory, independent body, at arm's length from the government, designed to monitor the performance of NHS Trusts, Primary Care Groups, local health groups and GP practices and to help secure quality improvement throughout the NHS in England and Wales. It was established as an integral part of the government's quality strategy described in the White Paper *The New NHS: Modern, Dependable* (DOH 1997) to enforce the clinical governance agenda. In effect, it will be a health service inspectorate in all but name, although it intends working with organisations in a facilitative and developmental way. It has statutory powers to enter NHS premises, gather information, copy records or databases and publish reports and is likely to become the most important force in the external review and monitoring of quality and performance in the NHS (Walshe 1999).

## Commissioning of healthcare

The way that the NHS ensures that the UK population has relevant health services available is through a commissioning process, based on local assessment of health need and the establishment of service level agreements to ensure that needs are met. This local work is currently the responsibility of the health authorities/health boards.

However, the organisation of the NHS is in the midst of structural change. The internal market, now abandoned, set health authorities/boards up as purchasers of services and hospitals, and community trusts as service providers. This purchaser/provider split was seen as preventing the component parts of the health services working in partnership for the benefit of the local population. The internal market and GP fundholding has been replaced by new ways of engaging groups of GPs and other primary care professionals in the commissioning of local services (see also PCGs, PCTs). The pace of change and the level of involvement of GPs in commissioning patient services varies considerably across the UK.

Each health authority is allocated a share of the resources available annually to commission all the services necessary for its registered or resident population. A national formula is used to identify an equitable share of the resources – this is called the capitation target. The formula takes into account the size, age distribution and health of the population, the level of social deprivation and the relative cost of building land and salaries.

## Community care

Responsibility for provision of care in the community has traditionally been divided between the Health Authorities and the social services. Following the change of government in May 1997, clear patterns have been emerging which are shaping the way community care will be delivered in the future. The NHS and local authorities are required to work together to enable as many people as possible to remain in their own homes and as far as possible maintain their independence. This policy relates to both older people and those with chronic illnesses and disabilities. For more detailed information see the government publications *Modernising Health and Social Services, National Priorities Guidance 1999/00–2001/02* (DOH 1998b) and *Better Services for Vulnerable People – Maintaining the Momentum* (DOH 1998c).

## Community and District Nursing Association

The Community and District Nursing Association (CDNA) is a specialist professional association and trades union representing community and district nurses. It is affiliated to the Trades Union Congress (TUC) and Scottish Trades Union Congress (STUC). It actively campaigns on issues of interest and concern to its members. ✉ ☎ ⌨

## Community Health Councils

Community Health Councils (CHCs) were established in 1974 by Act of Parliament, to represent the public interest in the NHS.

They existed across England and Wales and in Scotland are known as Health Councils. They had three main functions:

- representing public views
- monitoring and scrutinising the NHS
- providing complaints advice.

CHCs were member organisations with both rights and duties. There was usually at least one CHC for each local authority. CHCs also had regional and national bodies. The Association of Community Health Councils in England and Wales (ACHEW) (see below) had a team of staff who advised and provided member training.

CHC rights were:

- to receive information about local NHS services
- to be consulted about substantial changes in NHS services
- to comment on proposals affecting local services
- to access, by right, hospitals where NHS services are provided and, with permission, GP surgeries and other premises providing NHS services.

CHC duties were:

- to monitor local services
- to recommend improvements
- to hold an annual statutory meeting with the local Health Authority
- to produce an annual report
- to hold public meetings.

CHC members were nominated by local authorities and local voluntary organisations with some Secretary of State appointments. All CHC members were bound by their code of conduct and were required to declare any pecuniary interest. They were unpaid but were reimbursed expenses. They were required to represent the public, not their nominating body. Most NHS staff, and non-executive directors, were ineligible for membership because of the potential for a conflict of interests.

CHCs employed a small team, typically a chief officer and two or three other staff. Staff are employed by the NHS regional office but were independent of the local NHS.

CHC staff:

- provide information about local services, e.g. finding a doctor or dentist
- offer advice about local health and social services
- support those who wish to complain about NHS services
- advise CHC members.

CHC members:

- make visits to local hospitals to monitor services
- investigate local NHS services
- carry out surveys and research
- consider and comment on local and national NHS policy
- produce public reports on local NHS services
- attend Health Authority, NHS Trust and primary care group meetings to represent the public interest
- consult the public on substantial variations in local NHS services
- hold regular public meetings.

### Abolition of CHCs

In July 2000 the NHS National Plan for England (see National Plan) proposed the abolition of CHCs and the replacement of their functions by a range of bodies designed to promote 'citizen empowerment'. Although full details of the new bodies are not yet available, it appears that they will include a Patient Advocacy and Liaison Service (PALS) (see entry) and Patient Forums (see entry). The power to refer major planned changes to local NHS services to the Secretary of State will transfer to the scrutiny committees of local authorities. There will be a new Independent Reconfiguration Panel to deal with any appeals. Local authorities will also be given the power to scrutinise the local NHS and chief executives of local health organisations will be required to attend the scrutiny panel at least twice a year. At the time of writing, it appears that ACHEW (see below) and CHCs will be replaced by a national organisation called VOICE (see entry) and local organisations similarly named.

### Scotland and Northern Ireland

Local Health Councils undertake a similar role to CHCs and relate to Scottish Health Boards. In Northern Ireland, officers of the four health and social services councils perform the duties of the user representatives.

### 🔳 *The Association of Community Health Councils for England and Wales*

The Association of Community Health Councils for England and Wales (ACHEW) promoted CHC interests nationally and acted as a forum for discussion. It provided an information service and published a regular newsletter and briefing papers. ✉ ☽ 📄 🖰

## Community hospitals

Community hospitals are NHS hospitals providing intermediate care (see entry) for a local community. Care is managed by GPs, nurses and other therapists. Patients may receive all their necessary care in a community hospital for a period or may use it as a 'step-down' facility between an acute hospital episode and independent living at home or long-term care.

## 🔳 Community Hospitals Association

The Community Hospitals Association (CHA) exists to promote the improvements and extension of the range of services provided by community hospitals (see entry). Amongst other things it also collates and disseminates information on all aspects of work carried out in community hospitals; it demonstrates the quality and cost-effectiveness of community hospitals; it gives help to members in furthering the best interests of community hospitals; it supports them through periods of change; it promotes, assists and coordinates education and research; it promotes audit; it maintains a database; it encourages communication and it organises an annual symposium.

CHA is not to be confused with the Community Hospitals Group – a provider of independent hospital services in England. ✉ ☽ 📄 @ 🖰

## 🔳 Community Practitioners and Health Visitors Association

The Community Practitioners and Health Visitors Association (CPHVA) is the professional organisation for all community nursing and health visiting practitioners. It undertakes a range of education and training functions for its members. It is affiliated to Manufacturing Science and Finance (MSF). ✉ ☽

# Complaints

Used positively, the management of complaints can improve services and be a good learning experience for the professionals involved, as well as resulting in improved patient and client care. Regrettably, this is not always how complaints are perceived and all too often complainants are still faced with defensive and unhelpful responses which undermine public confidence in the health service. Much work is being done to improve the picture and a knowledge of the processes involved is essential for all healthcare professionals.

The NHS complaints procedure, in place since April 1996, applies, with only minor variations, across the whole of the UK. There are two levels at which complaints are made and handled – that of *local resolution* and that of *independent review*. Access to the Health Service Commissioner (more commonly known as the Ombudsman) is available for all of those who are not satisfied with the response they have received. NHS Trusts, Health Authorities and GPs must publicise their complaints procedures and must have a designated person to respond to complaints.

## *Local resolution*

There are a variety of possible stages. Ideally, complaints are dealt with and resolved as close to the source of complaint as possible, by the staff to whom the complaint is made. If that is not possible, then referral must be made to the relevant complaints manager. The Patient's Charter requires that a written complaint in a Trust receives a written reply by the Chief Executive. Health authorities would normally only become involved in a complaint made to a GP if local resolution has not been possible or if the individual chooses not to complain directly to the practice concerned. Set performance targets are in place for the speed at which replies must be dealt with.

## *Independent review panels*

These will be set up where local resolution has failed. The panel is set up as a committee of the Health Authority or Trust and is required to produce a confidential report setting out the results of its investigations, together with its conclusions and recommendations. The Chief Executive has to let the complainant know of any action taken by the Trust or Health Authority as a result of the panel report. Where a GP is involved, the Chief Executive of the Health Authority sends a copy of the report to the complainant. The GP has to let the complainant and the Health Authority know what action will be taken.

At either stage, complainants are informed of the roles and responsibilities of the Health Service Commissioner (Ombudsman), should they wish to pursue matters further.

## Complementary therapies

The inclusion of complementary therapies in mainstream health services often raises debates among clinical professionals. However, therapies such as reflexology, acupuncture and aromatherapy have now found a place in the NHS. They are offered by nurses, midwives, doctors, and members of the professions allied to medicine (PAMs). Complementary therapies can be broadly defined as being an addition to traditional care and treatment. 'Traditional' in this sense includes what it normally considered to be within the remit of modern western medicine. Although not all complementary therapies have their origins based in eastern or oriental medicine, they do not commonly originate from medicine as practised in Europe and North America, which owes much of its origins to the natural sciences which have been developed by western culture.

In establishing complementary therapies in the NHS, it is important to bear in mind that such therapies do not or should not be offered as a cure to a disease or condition. It needs to be emphasised that the prime purpose of complementary therapy is to assist patients/clients receiving treatment to experience fewer associated problems, or to make them feel better. For example, they can relieve nausea (notably for people receiving cytotoxic medication), relieve certain types of pain or induce wellbeing.

The question of vicarious liability has to be addressed when complementary therapies are offered. It is important that the organisations, such as hospitals, offering such therapies have a structure in place whereby the capabilities of practitioners offering a therapy can be checked, and that agreement is reached among other clinical professionals within the organisation, and that no false or misleading claims are ascribed to a therapy. If these safeguards are assured, there should be no reason why a

Trust or GP practice, for example, cannot offer complementary therapies tailored to the needs of a client group. It is important that any practitioners wishing to offer a complementary therapy must ensure that their professional leads are aware of their intention. After providing evidence of training and/or certification it would normally be necessary to ensure that the relevant manager and/or hospital committee had assessed the proposed therapy to ensure that it fits the aims and objectives of the Clinical Directorate or organisation. Once these assurances have been provided then it is possible to offer the therapy to patients, safe in the knowledge that they fully understand what the expected outcomes are and that this is appreciated equally by clinical colleagues who might otherwise raise objections.

## Confidentiality

All codes of conduct or ethics for the healthcare professions will address the issue of confidentiality in some way, at least in principle. Frequently, additional detailed advice is also available. All practitioners are expected to honour and respect the confidential information that they obtain in the course of their professional practice. Such information should not be disclosed to others without the patient's consent. Those who are being cared for have a right to expect that the information they disclose during the course of their care is kept confidential to those who are involved in their care. This is the basis of trust upon which care is given.

Information obtained during the course of professional practice should only be shared with others in exceptional circumstances. The principle of confidentiality should only be breached where disclosure is required by law or the order of a court, or is necessary in the public interest. The public interest can be interpreted as the interests of an individual, groups of individuals or society as a whole. The decision as to whether to disclose information must lie with the individual practitioner concerned and must be taken as a result of a considered assessment of all the relevant facts. The resultant decision should be recorded meticulously.

## Consent

This issue embodies the fundamental principle that every person has a right to choose what happens to him or her. Broadly, this can encompass both physical and psychological treatment, but is generally related to the giving of consent for physical invasive procedures.

This subject is covered by both criminal law (Offences against the Person Act 1861) and precedent set by the courts in civil cases. It is a basic rule of law that no-one has a right to touch another physically without consent. To do so would create the possibility of a claim for assault (an attempt to apply force to another, such as to put him or her in fear of physical violence) or battery (the actual application of physical force). The physical force does not have to be substantial and damage does not have to be caused, but intent to carry out the non-consensual contact must be present.

As the major legal defence against assault and battery is consent, the agreement of the patient must be sought before any physical treatment can be given by doctor or nurse. In practice, this often amounts to an informal verbal agreement between the patient and healthcare professionals, but in certain situations, e.g. when surgery is required, written consent to a specific treatment has to be obtained.

Consequently, the giving of consent is of paramount importance, and the law relating to this is strict. It is a legal requirement that an effective consent must satisfy the following criteria to ensure that it is a true consent (Carson & Montgomery 1991):

1. The patient must be able to understand the choices he or she is required to make.
2. Consent must be free and voluntary.
3. The procedure for which consent is sought must have been explained to the patient. It may be negligent to withhold important information.
4. Consent must not be produced by deceit.

To take account of the nature of medical and nursing practice, three exceptions to giving consent as above are acceptable but should be used with caution.

First, as outlined previously, an informal explanation and verbal agreement between patient and nurses is often sufficient to allow routine clinical care and treatment to be performed. This mainly involves care that the patient would normally carry out personally and excludes any medical intervention.

Second, the principle of 'necessity' will justify treatment of a patient where consent cannot be given, primarily in an emergency situation. As such, this exception permits life-saving treatment but should be applied in extreme situations only. The subsequent risk of a claim of assault and battery may be high if the patient would, in retrospect, have declined the treatment, or had previously expressed such a preference.

Third, and similarly to the above, an 'implied consent' can be relied upon if there is sufficient certainty that the patient would have requested or acceded to the treatment had it been offered in more controlled circumstances. Again, this applies to emergency events where either an initiation of a new treatment or an extension of an existing one is needed. In such events, it is ethically correct to consider that the treatment should be of obvious benefit to the patient, that it would be unreasonable to withhold it, and that no express objection has previously been given.

Children under 16 years of age can legally give their own consent if it is recognised that they have the capacity to understand what is involved and the consent is valid.

Relatives and close friends are frequently involved in care and consultation about patients, although they cannot in any situation legally give consent on behalf of the patient. This is governed by the legal rule that one adult does not have the authority to give consent for another adult. (Reproduced with kind permission from Weller 2000.)

## Consumer Health Information Centre

The Consumer Health Information Centre (CHIC) is an educational centre run by the Proprietary Association of GB, which is the trade association of all the companies and pharmaceuticals, etc. involved in over-the-counter medicines. It has a panel of health professionals and consumers and works with professional bodies to provide health information for the general public. An annual CHIC event is the colds and flu campaign which provides free leaflets and posters for pharmacies, health centres and doctors' surgeries.

## Consumer voices

Consumerism is the relationship and interaction that consumers have with businesses, government, public and private and

C

voluntary organisations. Consumerism within healthcare across the UK is complex and multifaceted, involving a range of people, organisations, structures and processes, both formal and informal. It has not developed specifically in relation to health but as part of the general consumer movement and the right to be heard. In both the public and independent healthcare sectors it has resulted in a shift of emphasis, away from individuals being in passive receipt of care to a more articulate, informed and demanding public who rightly expect quality care from healthcare professionals. Traditional professional attitudes and public subservience to the professions, particularly medicine, in part previously protected healthcare organisations from the wider consumer revolution which has been witnessed in other walks of life. A number of factors are now contributing to change, including:

- health consumer groups
- increased media involvement
- more accessible technology
- public sector and regulated health consumerism
- greater awareness of individual rights.

### Health consumer groups

A number of bodies are active in this field, including The Patient's Association which undertakes a major role as advocate on behalf of patients within the overall framework of healthcare consumerism. Established in1963, it is independent of government, health managers, professionals and the health industry. It exists to support individual patients to speak for themselves. Membership is on an individual basis and voluntary. Its philosophy is that the NHS is owned, used and paid for by the public and that everyone wants – and has the right – to be treated as a person, to be spoken to with kindness and understanding, and to be listened to carefully. The Association also reports regularly on private healthcare within the UK.

There are many other health consumer/patient information groups, many of which are disease specific, or orientated towards a particular clinical condition. Many exert considerable influence and may be consulted on health issues. Many of the more specific groups work alongside healthcare professionals in providing information and support for patients and their families, as well as being part of the general health consumer movement.

## Public sector health consumerism

Consumerism is formalised within the UK public sector through:

- patients' charters
- formal statutory mechanisms, e.g. Community Health Councils
- public participation in governance processes (e.g. Health Authority and Trust board membership)
- accessible complaints systems, active and formal government promotion of consumerism, standards of service and openness.

The Citizen's Charter of the early 1990s advanced consumerism in public services. Within the NHS, the Patient's Charter set out for the first time the standards and levels of service that patients could expect. Individual NHS Trusts were then required to develop their own charters. A new Patient's Charter is in preparation at the time of writing. Within health systems, statements of patients' and consumers' rights need to reflect the priorities and policies of the system. Consumerism in terms of the voice of the public forms part of the democratic electoral process within the UK. In addition, changes to UK health service legislation in the late 1990s aimed for:

- high quality and standards of care, accessible nationwide
- local responsibility in achieving these standards to ensure efficiency and value for money
- a partnership approach between health professional and the patient in determining service needs
- effective and open communication to rebuild public confidence in the NHS.

## Openness and consumerism in the NHS

Both NHS Health Authorities and Trusts are required to adhere to the Government's policy of openness and the NHS Code of Practice for Openness. This gives the public greater access to a wide range of information on activities and services within the NHS. Health Authorities must consult with CHCs and other interested parties on plans to change services and meetings must be open to the public. General practitioners are also required to provide practice leaflets regarding their services.

Consumers, as members of the public, can also become members of the Health Authorities and boards; this brings an element of consumerism to the overall framework of local health service governance.

## Contact a Family

Contact a Family (CAF) provides comprehensive information and helplines on over 300 self help groups dealing with rare disorders and medical conditions. They support the Rare Disorders Alliance and have a network of local groups throughout the country. ✉ ☎ 📄 @ 🔗

## Continuing professional development

Virtually all the healthcare professions have some form of continuing professional development (CPD) requirements, although they may be called by different names. A requirement to keep up to date with developments in one's own professional field is an integral part of being a professional and is usually enshrined in some form in the profession's code of conduct or similar. In addition, many professions increasingly impose statutory or mandatory requirements upon their practitioners in order for them to maintain registration or membership of their statutory or professional body. Advisory standards often also have a similar effect in practice as it is often difficult to obtain employment without having met certain professional development benchmarks.

The CPD requirements for each of the healthcare professions vary from profession to profession, and from time to time, and should be checked with the relevant standards-setting body for the individual profession. Two examples of different approaches to CPD are offered below.

### Nurses, midwives and health visitors

Each registered nurse, midwife and health visitor is required by law to:

- complete 5 days (or equivalent) of study activity every 3 years
- complete a notification of practice form

- use a personal professional profile
- undertake a return to practice programme after a break in practice of 5 years or more (see also PREP).

### Pharmacists

A pharmacist's responsibility to maintain competence and effectiveness as a practitioner is recognised in the Code of Ethics and Standards of Good Professional Practice within the *Medicines, Ethics and Practice: Guide to Pharmacists* (RPSGB 1997). The Royal Pharmaceutical Society of Great Britain has a 30 hour annual target for participation in continuing education (CE) for pharmacists. A national continuing education syllabus for pharmacy, together with sectoral syllabuses, for example, in industrial, veterinary and academic practice, is produced. Individuals are expected to cover the core and relevant sectoral syllabus/es every 5–8 years.

## COSHH regulations

The control of substances hazardous to health (COSHH) regulations 1988, amended 1998, introduced the concept of risk assessment in the workplace. Health hazards are categorised as 'irritant', 'corrosive', 'harmful', 'toxic', or 'very toxic'. Employers are obliged to assess substances against these criteria. Assessment also includes a description of the measures required to control the risks – whether that be by the elimination of the substances from the work process; containment within an enclosed system in order to prevent exposure; or safeguarding the individual with protective equipment or clothing. Continuous monitoring and review is required, including health surveillance and environmental monitoring. Scrupulous records must be kept. All health and safety law is enforced by The Health and Safety Executive (HSE).

## Council for Complementary and Alternative Medicines

Founded in 1985, the Council for Complementary and Alternative Medicines is committed to promoting and maintaining the highest standards of training, qualifications and treatment in complementary and alternative medicine. It provides a forum for communication and cooperation between the professional bodies representing acupuncture, medical herbalism, homeopathy and osteopathy. ✉ ☽ 🗎

## 🖾 Council for the Professions Supplementary to Medicine

The Council for the Professions Supplementary to Medicine (CPSM) is the statutory regulatory body which is responsible for maintaining the register for the professions supplementary to, or allied to, medicine (frequently collectively known as the PAMs). The CPSM sets the standards, controls and sanctions for these professions and has nearly 100 000 practitioners on its register. The CPSM was established in 1960 under the PSM Act 1960, but clause 47 of The Health Act 1997 repeals the 1960 PSM Act and establishes a new body known as the Health Professions Council (see entry), which it is anticipated will come into effect in September 2001. CPSM currently covers the professions of:

- art/drama/music and dance therapists
- chiropodists
- dietitians
- medical laboratory science officers
- occupational therapists
- prosthetists and orthotists
- physiotherapists
- orthoptists
- radiographers
- clinical scientists.

Speech and language therapists and paramedics are also on fast track for membership.

By separate statute, state registration is the criterion for employment in the professions in the NHS. Although not a requirement for private practice, state registration is considered to be the kite mark of quality in the individual professions, offering public protection.

The Council is run through a series of (currently) 7 boards representing the different professions; each board has an investigating and disciplinary committee and is charged with producing a code of conduct. The majority of members of each board are directly elected and a minority appointed from the Medical Royal Colleges, universities, employers and other special interest groups. Each board elects a practising member of the profession to the Council. The remaining members of the Council and boards are appointed by the government departments, medical Royal Colleges, educational interests and the GMC. The Council chairman is appointed by the privy council but each board elects its own chairman from amongst its own profession. ✉ ① ▤

## Credit Accumulation and Transfer Schemes

Often a source of confusion to the uninitiated Credit Accumulation and Transfer Schemes (CATS) and APL/APEL (see entry) are frequently referred to together. They are actually separate processes, either of which may take place separately or they may be linked together in practice.

In CATS, *credit* is the unit of 'currency' used in education, awarded either retrospectively for work which has already been undertaken, or attached to academic study currently being undertaken. A certain number of credits, at certain levels, constitute different types of academic awards. For example, in England 360 credits are needed for a first degree (honours). In a modular programme, a student chooses from a variety of modules which will have different credit ratings, in order to work toward the acquisition of a diploma or degree. The same principles apply elsewhere in the UK, for example, Scotland's SCOT-CAT system, although the amount of credit will vary, reflecting the differences in the higher education system in place. Credit is therefore *accumulated* in pursuit of one's eventual goal. In theory, credit can also be *transferred* – either to another programme within the same institution, or to another institution. The reality is not always as easy, as there are no national credit schemes yet in place, although these have been talked about for some time. The principles underlying credit schemes are to ensure that students do not duplicate learning already achieved and that all study of an appropriate level and depth is rewarded.

APL and APEL – often written as AP(E)L – refers to the Assessment of Prior (Experiential) Learning. The learning can either have been certificated in some way (APL) or can be from experience (hence experiential) (APEL). An individual, therefore, who is in pursuit of a particular qualification can ask to have previous relevant learning taken into account, or credited – perhaps from a course or courses they may have undertaken, or from experience. Clearly the learning has to be demonstrable and this can be done in a number of ways – through the use of portfolios of learning, the writing of assignments or the presentation of case studies, for example. AP(E)L processes are time consuming for those involved and because they are resource intensive, can be expensive, although the actual cost varies from institution to institution.

# A–Z guide

## Data Protection Act 1984

The Data Protection Act gives patients and clients access to their computer held records. It also regulates the storage and protection of patient and client information held on computer. The system for dealing with applications for access is set out in the *Access to Health Records Act 1990: a Guide for the NHS* published by the government health departments (DOH 1990). All healthcare practitioners must be aware of and honour the rights of patients and clients on this issue.

## Dental bodies corporate

Throughout the 20th century the vast majority of dental treatment in the UK was provided by dentists working single handed or in group dental practices. However, at the beginning of the new millennium a new trend in the provision of dental healthcare is emerging.

Dental bodies corporate (DBCs) are companies which are registered with the General Dental Council (GDC) and as such are permitted to carry on the business of dentistry. Since 1995, legislation has not allowed the creation of new DBCs and therefore the 27 companies currently registered with the GDC represent an exclusive club. In the last 10 years there has been an explosion in corporate dentistry culminating in the purchase of DBCs by Boots the Chemist plc in 1998 and the opening of four Boots Dental Care Practices in 1999. Integrated Dental Holdings, currently the largest chain, already has some 70 practices and employs several hundred dentists. Various competitors are moving in the same direction. The purchase price of a shell DBC has reputedly increased from approximately £10 000 10 years ago to almost £150 000 now, reflecting the commercial importance of this trend.

The dental profession as a whole is watching these developments with considerable interest and, in some quarters, scepticism. The DBCs have access to venture capital and their purchasing power and increasing political influence are having a significant impact in the dental world. It remains to be seen whether the dental practices of old survive into the next century although there seems little doubt that DBCs are here to stay.

**D**

## Department of Health, England

The Department of Health (DOH) is responsible for promoting and protecting the health of the nation, providing a National Health Service in England and providing social care including the overseeing of personal social services run by local authorities in England. The Department represents UK health policy interests in the EU and through relevant international organisations including WHO. It also supports UK based healthcare and pharmaceutical industries. (See also DHSS Northern Ireland, Scottish Parliament and Welsh Assembly.) ✉ ☎ 🖐

## Department of Health and Social Services, Northern Ireland

The Department of Health and Social Services (DHSS) is responsible for securing an integrated service promoting the health and welfare of the population through three main programmes: health and personal social services, social security and child maintenance. It is responsible for hospitals, family practitioner services and community health and for the administration of the health and personal and social services working through the four area health boards which purchase health and social services for their populations. The Department also has responsibility for health promotion and certain elements of social legislation and administration. The impact of the new Northern Ireland Assembly upon the current arrangements is not yet clear. ✉ ☎

## Department for International Development

The Department for International Development (DFID) is part of the Foreign and Commonwealth Office responsible for the UK's overseas aid to developing countries, for global environmental assistance and for assistance to Central and Eastern Europe and the former Soviet Union. The DFID works in partnership with developing countries through their respective governments, international organisations and non-governmental organisations. It concentrates particularly on improving standards of health and healthcare for people in developing countries, particularly women and children. Work is done to reduce the spread of serious communicable diseases like malaria, TB and measles and to help women avoid unwanted pregnancies and sexually transmitted diseases. ✉ ☽

## Devolution

The elections that took place in the UK in May 1999 led to devolution of power, in relation to the provision of health and social care, from central UK government in Westminster to Scotland, Northern Ireland and Wales. Management of the NHS is carried out via the NHS Executive in the Department of Health in England, the NHS Management Executive in the Scottish Executive Health Department in Scotland, the NHS Directorate in Wales and the Health and Personal Social Services Management Group in the Department of Health, Social Services and Public Safety in Northern Ireland.

## Distance Learning see Open Learning

### Education consortia see Workforce planning

### EEC/EU directives

These are a form of European legislation (see European Union) which have relevance to the healthcare professions. There are two types of EU directives – sectoral and general systems.

*Sectoral directives* have been achieved for specific professions by a process known as harmonisation. They have come about as a result of work on the part of the relevant profession, working through an Advisory Committee in Brussels, to agree minimum standards for the profession concerned in relation to education and qualifications. The purpose of such an activity is to allow freedom of movement of members of that profession within the EU. Doctors, dentists, GPs, midwives, nurses responsible for general care, pharmacists and veterinary surgeons all have specific sectoral directives.

*General system directives* are directives based on the principle of recognition, not harmonisation. They came about because the process of harmonisation took such a long time – for example, the architects' sectoral directive took 17 years to produce. No conditions for training are stipulated in the sectoral directives but the applicants' qualifications are assessed by the designated authority in the host country. Any shortfall in training or experience may have to be made up before the individual is eligible to register his or her qualification in the UK. Within the health field this is the route used by those professions without sectoral directives – for example, a physiotherapist trained in France who wishes to work in the UK would apply to the CPSM (see entry) as the designated authority to assess his or her qualifications.

Moves are currently afoot, under an initiative known as simpler legislation for the internal market (SLIM), to simplify the existing legislation which allows freedom of movement within the European Union. The approach is to devolve more power and responsibility to the individual professions and to reduce the input and involvement of the European Commission. Whether this approach is in order to accord more authority to the professions or is merely a way of saving the Commission money is a matter of debate.

## Electronic records

Electronic records fall into two categories:

- electronic *patient* records – the information held (and ideally shared) by different health professionals and health organisations about a patient
- electronic *health* records, containing a summary of an individual's key health details.

The development of electronic records is an important aspect of the Government's information for health strategy (DOH 1998c), and since April 2000, four large-scale, DOH-funded pilot schemes have been working to develop and implement shared electronic record systems across health and social services. The Electronic Records Development and Implementation Programme (http://www.nhsia.nhs.uk/erdip/) focuses on various aspects of the development of electronic records in healthcare. Confidentiality and security, technical standards and professional standards for using electronic records are currently under development. By 2005, electronic patient records are to be accessible for 24-hour emergency care and personal electronic health records are to be implemented at primary care level. (See also: DOH 1998c (http://www.doh.gov.uk/nhsexipu/whatnew/ehrdis.htm).)

## Emotional intelligence

This is a term, coined in the USA, which has been described as the ability and intent to make one's emotions work for one, either personally or in the workplace, by acknowledging their contribution to behaviours and thinking. This might sound straightforward, but it needs to be considered in the context of the workplace of the last decades of the last century, where scientific proof is deemed to be required before anything done has credibility. The drive towards evidence based practice is ensuring that this is becoming even more the case in the NHS. However, there are some instances in both personal and professional life where it can be helpful to acknowledge and use feelings. Weisinger (2000) cites the work of Mayer and Salovey, who coined the term 'emotional intelligence' in 1990, and describes four stages to developing emotional intelligence:

1. developing the ability to accurately perceive, appraise and express emotion
2. developing the ability to access or generate feeling on demand when that can help you to understand your own feelings or those of another person
3. developing the ability to understand emotions and the knowledge that you can derive from them
4. developing the ability to regulate emotions to promote emotional and intellectual growth. (Weisinger 2000)

In this context, the term *emotion* is used in the broadest psychological sense, to encompass feelings of all types, rather than in the more generalist interpretation of emotion as something which is distressing, and which may compromise judgement.

## Empowerment

To empower means to enable and is a popular term used by many disciplines to explain the process of granting power to self and others. In healthcare, over the last decade it has become a common 'buzz' word, which in organisational terms is deemed to be a good thing. Empowerment is described from two perspectives in healthcare – empowerment as it relates to the individual and empowerment in organisations.

### Empowerment as it relates to the individual

According to Gibson (1991) empowerment is a social process of recognising, promoting and enhancing individuals' ability to meet their own needs, solve their own problems and mobilise the necessary resources. This leads to a feeling of being in control of one's own life.

This approach implies that individuals take control of their own lives and accept responsibility for their own action and behaviours. Hopson and Scally (1981) point out that many people do not believe they own their life or growth or development.

They often work and live in environments that by design or by accident leave them with little power. Disempowerment is the result of believing that nothing can be done to change the situation and rendering oneself dependent on others.

Following a systematic review of the literature, Hokanson Hawkes (1992) concluded that the environment is significant in ensuring empowerment can succeed for the individual. There needs to be trust, open and honest communication, mutual respect, courtesy, acceptance of people and valuing of others.

### Empowerment in organisations

Whether in hospital, community setting or classroom, empowerment is an essential component for personal growth and development. Manthey (1994) suggests that people need to know what is expected of them and what the limits are if they are to be in control of their decision making. A simple model, clarifying levels of responsibility, authority and accountability, is helpful in ensuring individuals are clear about what is expected of them. She suggests that in a typical change management scenario it is important to associate the level of authority for the decision with the level of the issue being discussed.

As organisations flatten, decisions are made at lower levels. For people to feel that they are in control they need to be aware of the decision-making boundaries. This leads to avoidance of blame, promotes and encourages effective relationship management and creates an environment of risk taking.

Individual empowerment leads to organisational empowerment that is achieved, according to Exley (1993), when staff understand the goals of the organisation, their role in relation to the goal achievement and have the opportunity to learn and develop new skills.

Such findings are of considerable relevance within the context of the health services, particularly when applied to the recruitment, retention and overall management of staff.

## English National Board for Nursing, Midwifery and Health Visiting

The English National Board for Nursing, Midwifery and Health Visiting (ENB) is a non-departmental government body which fulfils the statutory functions set out in the Nurses, Midwives and Health Visitors Act 1979 and its subsequent amendments. Its main purpose is to ensure that the institutions it approves conduct educational programmes which equip nurses, midwives and health visitors to meet existing and changing healthcare needs. The ENB currently has 10 members, 3 executives and 7 non-executives nominated by the Secretary of State. Following a government review, all 4 national boards and the UKCC are due to be replaced by a new UK statutory regulatory body to be called the Nurses and Midwives Council. National arrangements will vary but plans are being made for the ENB to move into the NHS Executive in Leeds as an Education and Training Unit. (See also National Board for Nursing, Midwifery and Health Visiting for Scotland (NBS), National Board for Nursing, Midwifery and Health Visiting for Northern Ireland (NBNI), United Kingdom Central Council for Nursing, Midwifery and Health Visiting (UKCC) and Welsh National Board (WNB).) ✉ ☾ 📄 ✎

## ▧ Equal Opportunities Commission

The Equal Opportunities Commission (EOC) exists to challenge discrimination, champion equality and act as a catalyst for change. Their vision is a society that enables men and women to fulfil their potential and have their contributions to work and home life equally valued and respected, and free from assumptions based on their sex. ✉ ☾ @ ✎

## Ethics

All healthcare professionals need an understanding of the concepts and underpinning principles of ethics and its application to their daily work. An enormous subject in its own right, time and space allow only a brief discussion here.

Knowledge informing healthcare requires to be accurate and where possible established on sound research evidence. Skilled interventions based on such knowledge must be performed safely and effectively. In essence, there is a right and wrong way to influence healthcare.

There is a dimension of 'right' and 'wrong' linking these concepts with perceived degrees of goodness. This is the moral or ethical dimension of healthcare (Edwards 1996, Johnston 1994). The concern is thus with what one ought or ought not to do in particular circumstances. The question 'how do I keep this patient alive?' is an issue resolved by addressing knowledge problems and applying skilled interventions. Conversely, the question 'should I keep this patient alive?' invites questions of doing what is good or morally right. Health professionals confront such moral dilemmas daily.

In general, ethics is characterised by distinct orientations. Within the *teleological* perspective, a term denoting consequences, the ethical position is valued in accordance with anticipated outcomes. This position is mainly presented in *utilitarian* ethics wherein the principle of right is that which leads to good, specifically the greatest good for the greatest number. The *deontological* perspective, a term dealing with duty derived from intrinsic value, adjudges an act as being right or wrong because it is intrinsically or self evidently good, that is, it is always wrong to deliberately kill or let die, irrespective of wider consequences. The teleological or utilitarian viewpoint may argue that dropping a nuclear bomb on Hiroshima is justified because whilst thousands would be killed, hundreds of thousands, perhaps millions, would be saved by shortening the war. The deontological viewpoint may claim that outcome arguments could never justify killing innocent people.

Of consequence is the means of arriving at ethical decisions. One viewpoint is that universal rules or principles guide moral decisions. Of significance is the perspective within biomedical ethics known as the 'four principles' approach (Beauchamp & Childress 1994). These four principles are:

- beneficence – doing good
- non-maleficence – doing no harm
- autonomy – respecting individuals' choice
- justice – making fair and equitable decisions.

Situation ethics (Fletcher 1966) by contrast, argues that it is not possible to apply universal principles – moral dilemmas are contextualised within social situations and resolved through dialogue and reflection; someone who responds to ethical problems by rigidly following rules or principles is not a free moral agent.

The differing voice encountered within womens' literature and scholarly studies is articulated in the dynamic of an ethic of care (Gilligan 1982, Noddings 1984). The call to care and to responsibility invokes a compassionate intent to do good. Thus, caring is intrinsically ethical; to care is to live ethically. It is a way of being in which caring is deemed an ethical virtue, aligning the perspective with virtue ethics.

## European Union

The European Union (EU) is a grouping of member states committed to economic, social and political integration. It has widespread ramifications for all aspects of life for those in the member states but only those issues with relevance to health will be dealt with here.

Current member states are Austria, Belgium, Denmark, Finland, France, Germany, Greece, Ireland, Italy, Luxembourg, the Netherlands, Portugal, Spain, Sweden and the UK. The European Economic Area (EEA) is a wider grouping of EU countries, with the addition of Iceland and Norway. Bulgaria, Cyprus, the Czech Republic, Estonia, Hungary, Latvia, Lithuania, Malta, Poland, Romania, Slovakia and Slovenia are all currently seeking membership of the EU.

### Institutions of the EU

#### European Parliament
Established in 1979 the European Parliament, sitting in Strasbourg and Brussels, is currently composed of 567 elected members (MEPs) who are grouped by political affiliation, rather than nationality. The UK currently has 87 members and elections take place every 5 years. The Parliament has an input into the EC's budget and amends and vetoes laws on the single market, education, training, consumer rights, the arts and health.

#### Council of Ministers
The Council of Ministers is the main legislative arm of the EU and has the final say on adopting EU law. The Council of Ministers consists of one minister from each of the member states with participating ministers varying according to the issue under discussion. It meets in private and its presidency rotates every 6 months between member states in alphabetical order. The Council's role is to examine draft legislation drawn up by the EC and amend, accept or reject it.

### The European Commission

The European Commission (EC) has a political, technical and judicial role. It is responsible for drafting proposals for EU legislation. It is the EU's executive body and civil service and can issue regulations of its own accord (see below). The 17 commissioners are nominated by the governments of the member states and are bound by oath to act independently of those governments in the interests of the EU as a whole. Commissioners work in 22 different departments known as Directorates General (DGs). The Directorates of particular interest to the healthcare professions are DGI (External Relations); DGIII (Internal Market and Industrial Affairs); and DGV (Employment, Industrial Relations and Social Affairs).

**E**

### Court of Justice

Based in Luxembourg, the Court of Justice consists of 13 judges from the member states assisted by the Advocate-General. The rulings of the courts are final in matters of European Law which take precedence over national law.

### *European Union Legislation*

There are four main types of EU legislation.

### Regulation

A regulation has direct legal force in the member states although it may in certain cases mean changes to national law. Regulations are principally used for decisions with immediate effect.

### Directive

A directive sets out the principles of legislation but leaves it to each member state to implement it through national law. The Council of Ministers agrees a time limit for this to be done which is normally 2–3 years. In the UK, EU legislation is frequently implemented through a statutory instrument laid before Parliament under the European Communities Act. In some cases the new law is incorporated in a draft bill which amends existing national legislation. If the provisions of the directive are already covered by an existing Act of Parliament then no further action is needed. (See EEC Directives.)

### Decision

A decision, issued by the Council of Ministers, is a law binding only on those member states, companies or individuals to whom it is addressed.

### Recommendation

A recommendation or opinion is a statement, not a law, and neither is binding on member states.

## Evidence-based practice

Clinical judgement together with the best available evidence makes for evidence-based practice (EBP). Information and flows of information throughout the world have had a real impact in the way decisions are made. Results of treatment may be compared, not only with the hospital next door, but potentially with the hospital on the other side of the world. Technology has increased the availability of research findings and the growth of a research culture in the health services has increased the amount of research being carried out. The combination of these two factors plus a healthcare context characterised by increasing consumer awareness, cost pressures, professional self-regulation and clinical governance have created an environment in which a commitment to achieving EBP has grown.

The term evidence based practice is a synthesis of the terminology of science and professional practice: science, because the term 'evidence based' implies the concept of scientific rationality, and professional practice, because it is about individual practitioner behaviour (Lockett 1997). EBP is a process. It is about finding, appraising and then applying best available evidence to the treatment and management of healthcare. The main purpose of implementing EBP should be to improve care for patients. It does this by supporting the practitioners in their decision making. This enables practitioners to commit themselves to a systematic approach to practice development.

There are a number of models for developing EBP, such as reflective practice, role modelling, action learning groups, research awareness groups and clinical supervision. All these approaches ensure that a balance is struck between scientific findings and the personal experience of practitioners working with clients.

On an organisational level, four areas were identified by Walsh and Ham (1997) as being particularly important in achieving EBP:

- a scientific culture – emphasising the importance of systematic enquiry, moving away from purely opinion based activity
- managing knowledge – to have systems in place that make seeking, finding and disseminating knowledge easy
- systems for change – the formal use of systems such as audit and care pathways for critically analysing the quality of care
- incentive to change – understanding how and why practitioners change and making sure that systems encourage positive changes.

Achieving EBP is a worthy goal both for individual practitioners and for the wider healthcare arena. It is complex and multifaceted and by its very definition always changing and never entirely achievable.

The ability to deliver EBP is a key requirement of professional practice. In order to do this, it is important that the individual professional is able to interpret for him or herself the robustness and integrity of the evidence as presented. It is not sufficient to accept that research processes which have resulted in the evidence being published are robust just because they have been published. It remains the individual responsibility of each practitioner to satisfy him or herself that the processes have been appropriately applied. In order that they may do this, individuals need to be familiar with the characteristics of a number of research paradigms, and their methodological approaches. In this way, practitioners can satisfy themselves that the researchers have adhered to the principles and processes of good research practice.

The National Institute for Clinical Excellence (NICE), is there to help health professionals in that its guidelines have been prepared after the underpinning research has been scrutinised by a team of experienced people. However, it remains the responsibility of each professional to ensure that he or she administers the correct treatment to patients, and thus to do this safely, professionals should ensure that they understand the underlying research processes.

## Family Planning Association see fpa

### fpa

The fpa, previously known as The Family Planning Association, is the only registered charity working to improve sexual health and reproductive rights of all people throughout the UK. It works with the public and professionals to ensure high quality information and services are available for everyone who needs them. It offers advice on a range of issues including contraception, abortion, sexually transmitted diseases and sexual health in general. ✉ ☎ ⌂

## Freedom of Information Act

The Freedom of Information (FOI) Act allows every individual or organisation the right to see government and public service documents of any kind. It is a very powerful tool for undertaking government and public policy research.

# A–Z guide

## General Dental Council

The General Dental Council (GDC) is the statutory regulatory body for dentists. The first Dentists Act was passed in 1878 and initiated the registration of dentists. The current legislation is the Dentists Act 1984. The GDC has three main functions:

- setting standards for the registration, professional education, professional conduct and fitness to practice of dentists
- preventing those who are not qualified from practising dentistry
- the regulation of dental auxiliaries.

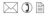

## General Medical Council

The General Medical Council (GMC) is the statutory regulatory body for doctors in the UK and licenses doctors to practise medicine in the UK. It was established in 1853 and currently works within the remit of the Medical Act 1983. It works to protect patients and to guide doctors through its legislation which requires the GMC to:

- keep up-to-date registers of qualified doctors
- foster good medical practice
- promote high standards of medical education
- deal firmly and fairly with doctors whose fitness to practice is in doubt.

There are currently about 189 000 names on the medical register. Doctors are eligible for registration if they:

- qualify at a UK medical school
- qualify elsewhere in the EEA and are EEA nationals
- qualify at certain recognised medical schools outside the EEA.

Limited registration, allowing practice under supervision, is available for those qualifying elsewhere.

There are currently 104 members of the GMC consisting of:

- 54 doctors elected by doctors on the register
- 25 members of the public (not medically qualified) nominated by the privy council
- 25 doctors appointed by education bodies – the universities, the medical Royal Colleges and faculties.

✉ ① 📄 ⌐

## G

## ▨ General Optical Council

The General Optical Council is the statutory regulatory body for the optical profession in the UK. Opticians are broadly organised into two branches: *optometrists* (*or ophthalmic opticians*) who undertake the testing of sight and eye examinations and usually fit and supply optical appliances; and *dispensing opticians* who fit and supply optical appliances but do not test sight.

Registration with the Council is required by law if an individual wishes to practise as an optician. The relevant legislation is The Opticians Act 1989 which consolidates the 1959 Act of the same name and its amending legislation. ✉ ① 📄

## ▨ General Osteopathic Council

The General Osteopathic Council (GOsC) was established as a result of the Osteopaths Act 1993, when osteopathy became the first of the complementary medical professions to achieve statutory self-regulation. Its remit is to: 'provide for the regulation of the professions of osteopathy including the registration of osteopaths and their professional education and conduct and for promotion and development of the profession'. The Council has 6 lay members, 1 Secretary of State appointee, 3 education members and 12 osteopathic members. ✉ ① 📄

## General Practitioner services

General practitioners in the UK are independent contractors who provide services through contracts of service held with the NHS. As such, they are not employees of the NHS, but self-employed professionals, a significant number of whom work as partners in group practices. Included in the ranks of general practitioners are:

- 30 000 family doctors or GPs
- 15 000 dentists

- 11 000 opticians
- 10 000 retail pharmacists.

From 1948, contracts for these practitioners were administered by organisations directly responsible to the Ministry of Health. Initially, these organisations were called Executive Committees, subsequently renamed as Family Practitioner Committees in 1974, then renamed Family Health Services Authorities (FHSAs) in 1991. The essential functions of these had been:

- to assess the health needs of their local population
- to maintain a register of patients on GP lists
- to reimburse practitioners for work done
- to assess the needs of the local population
- to develop services in collaboration with other health authorities and GPs
- to investigate complaints relating to breaches of the contracts of service
- to implement health policies as issued by the DOH.

In 1996, FHSAs and District Health Authorities (DHAs) were amalgamated, thereby unifying the health authorities' purchasing, planning and monitoring functions.

GPs had previously been paid by a combination of capitation fee (i.e. based on the number of patients on the GP's list) and a number of fees for items of service. GPs were also entitled to claim reimbursement for practice expenses such as renting of premises, employment of receptionists, cleaning, heating, and lighting. In 1990, new contract terms were introduced, including 'target payments'.

The GP services have been the traditional area where successive governments have introduced charges. Currently, charges are collected from patients for the following:

- each item on GP prescriptions
- eye tests and dispensing of spectacles
- dental care received.

## General Social Care Council

The General Social Care Council (GSCC) is the new statutory regulatory body being established for social care staff. It will replace the Council for the Education and Training of Social Work (CETSW). It will be responsible for setting standards for education, registration, conduct and practice and will maintain a register of those working in social care. It will draw up a code of practice for employers, to be enforced by the Regional Commission for Care Standards. Initially, registration will be restricted to qualified social workers and residential child care staff.

## Genetic engineering

This is an umbrella term used for the manipulation of the genes of plants and animals. Genes can be transplanted between widely different species to create characteristics which the host would not have in its natural state. Gene therapy is a technique whereby a missing or faulty gene is replaced so that the body can control or cure disease. Whilst there is evidence that such activity can be of great benefit to patients, for example, in the administration of the healthy gene to those with cystic fibrosis via a nasal spray, the ethical implications of such potential activity are immense for all healthcare professionals. There are also numerous other ramifications which have yet to be fully explored and the debate looks set to continue for years to come.

## Genetic Interest Group

The Genetic Interest Group (GIG) is a national alliance representing individuals and families affected by genetic disorders. It has over 100 voluntary organisations in membership and its primary aims are to increase public awareness of genetic disorders and to improve services for people affected by them. ✉ ☽ 📄 @ ✎

## Green Papers

The term Green Paper refers to a government report which contains proposals for discussion and consultation. Green Papers are frequently followed by White Papers, although White Papers are not necessarily preceded by Green Papers.

## Grey letter

The term 'grey letter' refers to a proposal from the NHS Executive made in 1999 which could result in a planned alert letter being sent to trusts and health authorities naming practitioners from any discipline who have been sacked or suspended and may represent a risk to patients. The criteria for a letter being sent are '...that the employee is a potential danger to patients, as identified for example by suspension, dismissal or police investigation, and it is considered that the individual may seek employment in health or social care elsewhere either permanently or as a locum either in an NHS hospital or elsewhere'. The types of offence which may result in such action might include:

- indecent assault
- fraud or theft
- poor professional performance
- health problems
- unwillingness to accept constructive criticism and retraining
- being reported to a disciplinary body e.g. GMC, UKCC.

During consultation this measure was strongly attacked as an infringement of an individual's rights by the unions. Concern has been expressed particularly in relation to the absence of criteria for the removal or cancellation of a grey letter and the effect unproven allegations may have on an individual's career. There is real concern that the proper role of the regulatory bodies could be undermined by such an initiative as they attempt to put steps in place to deal with poor performance. Other significant concerns are that the use of such letters could breach some articles of the European Convention on Human Rights and European Community law of data processing.

## Your Guide to the NHS

Published in 2000, *Your Guide to the NHS* sets out not only what patients can expect from the NHS, as described in the NHS Plan (see entry), but also the responsibilities which are expected of patients, for example, in terms of cancelling appointments if they cannot be met.

## Health

Health is frequently defined objectively. We also sometimes feel it is readily recognised subjectively, particularly when we encounter its absence. But the task of defining what is essentially an experiential phenomenon is difficult, and the mere absence of clearly discernible signs and symptoms of illness does not necessarily confirm the presence of health.

In increasing our understanding of the concept we do need a starting point. On a reductionist interpretation, health might be defined as simply as the absence of disease. The World Health Organisation (WHO) at its inception, offered the definition of health as a state of complete physical, mental and social well-being and not merely the absence of disease or infirmity (WHO 1946). This provoked a more meaningful interpretation. However, this definition is problematic in a number of regards. First, there is the problem of establishing the meaning of wellbeing. Some people may achieve high levels of experiential wellbeing (which might be defined as the feel-good factor) while suffering some degree of biological disease or infirmity. Others may be functioning adequately physically, mentally and socially but still not experience such levels of life satisfaction. Indeed, Downie (1990) has suggested that, while health and wellbeing may overlap as states of being, they are distinct concepts. On another level, the WHO definition is criticised as being idealistic: does anyone have complete physical, mental and social wellbeing at all times? In this respect Antonovsky (1996) has suggested that we are all somewhere between the imaginary poles of total wellness and total illness. Finally, it is suggested (Downie et al 1990) that in referring only to physical, mental and social aspects, the definition ignores other aspects such as emotional and spiritual wellbeing.

All this highlights the point that, as suggested by Seedhouse (1986), health means different things to different people. On this basis, he claims that a personal optimum state of health is equivalent to the state of the set of conditions which fulfil or enable a person to work to fulfil his or her realistic chosen and biological potential. This recognition of the contextual nature of health was already affirmed by WHO (1984) in its own description of health in terms of:

> The extent to which an individual or group is able, on the one hand, to realise aspirations and satisfy needs and on the other hand, to change or cope with the environment. Health is therefore seen as a resource for everyday life, not an object of living: it is a positive concept emphasising social and personal resources as well as physical capabilities.

According to Slevin (1999) there are two significant aspects of such conceptualisations: health is embedded in social contexts and rests to a large extent on aspirations for quality of life; and the capacity for change and willingness to make changes are fundamental to each person's evolving commitment to health. On this basis, concepts of health and health promotion cannot be imposed but emerge through empowering dialogue and negotiation.

## The Health Act 1999

This Act came into force on 5 July 1999 in England. It implements the proposals in the English White Paper *The New NHS: Modern, Dependable* (DOH 1997). It marks the end of NHS competition, ends fundholding and requires doctors, nurses, trusts and health authorities to cooperate. It gives primary care trusts a legal status. Its main provisions include:

- the abolition of GP fundholding
- local healthcare driven by health improvement programmes
- powers to remove barriers between the NHS, social services and wider local government
- high security hospitals may become NHS Trusts
- the creation of the Commission for Health Improvement as a statutory body

- a statutory duty on all NHS Trusts to improve the quality of care
- reserve powers to support the pharmaceutical price regulation scheme, by which the price of drug charges to the NHS is monitored and controlled
- NHS tribunals to have new powers to disqualify doctors and other health practitioners who commit fraudulent acts or who act in ways detrimental to the health service
- new powers to the Secretary of State to monitor professional competence
- new patient service partnerships, such as walk in centres.

## Health Action Zones

The term Health Action Zones (HAZs) describes the initiative to bring together NHS, local government organisations and others to develop and implement a locally agreed strategy for improving the health of the local people as part of a 'seamless service'. Activity is driven and coordinated by individual health authorities. They are part of the government's initiative to reduce health inequalities and prevent illness in those areas with high levels of poor health and deprivation. First announced in principle in 1997, they went live in April 1999. Initiatives cover a range of issues such as drug problems, smoking cessation and teenage health problems.

## Health Advisory Service

Established as the Hospital Advisory Service in 1975, the organisation has undergone a number of changes since its inception. Its current role is:

- to advise on the maintenance and improvement of the standard of management, organisation and delivery of patient care services, mainly those for mentally ill and elderly people
- to publish general guidance, based on service reviews, for the use of health and local authorities and to issue an annual report
- to keep government aware of the standards of service provision for the client groups concerned
- to identify problem areas in the provision of services, especially those that may need to be addressed by changes of policy or its implementation

- to identify good practices and to disseminate them and encourage their adoption. ✉ ➀ 🖹

## Health Authorities

Until 2002, Health Authorities served populations of about 500 000 and had a range of responsibilities, including:

- assessing the health needs of the local population
- developing a Health Improvement Programme (see entry) to meet those needs in partnership with other key players
- purchasing hospital and community, including primary care, services for the local population within financial allocations
- monitoring services provided by Trusts and ensuring charter standards are achieved
- developing plans for health services in conjunction with other bodies, e.g. local authorities and voluntary organisations.

(*See* Strategic Health Authorities.)

## ▨ Health Coalition Initiative

The Health Coalition Initiative (HCI) is a partnership network for voluntary health organisations, pharmaceutical companies and health and information professionals. HCI aims to build bridges between patients and their carers, pharmaceutical companies and the NHS by facilitating multidisciplinary discussions on current issues in a rapidly changing healthcare environment. ✉ ➀ 🖹 @

## ▨ Health Education Authority

The Health Education Authority (HEA) was a key source of health promotion in England until its abolition in 2000. It was a special health authority within the NHS. It advised government and undertook research, consultation and policy developments in support of national health promotion campaigns. Areas of work included, for example, accidents, alcohol, primary health care, professional development, mental health and nutrition. It worked within the public and private sectors, both nationally and internationally. It offered a range of services including: research, monitoring and evaluation of health trends, strategic planning and policy developments for government, professional standards and development, publications, international technical assistance, a library, and events and conferences. ✉ ➀

## ◧ Health Education Board for Scotland

The Health Education Board for Scotland (HEBS) gives leadership to the health education effort in Scotland by:

- ensuring that people have adequate information about health and the factors which influence it
- helping people to acquire the motivation and skills which enable them to safeguard their own health and other people's health
- promoting commitment to, and participation in, health promotion at all levels of society
- encouraging and enabling policy makers at all levels to recognise possible health consequences of their activities and to make policies which promote health.

## Health for All

In May 1981, the World Health Assembly, the governing body of WHO, which meets annually in Geneva, adopted a global strategy in support of Health for All by the year 2000. Its goal is the attainment by all citizens of the world of a level of health that will permit them to lead a socially and economically productive life. Primary health care is seen as the key to achieving the objective through initiatives such as safe water, immunisation, local healthcare and trained local personnel to attend childbirth.

## Health Improvement Programmes

Health improvement programmes (HImPs) are action programmes to improve health and healthcare locally led by the Health Authority. The programmes will involve Trusts, primary care groups and other primary care professionals, working in partnership with the local authority and engaging other local interests. The intention is that each Health Authority should have a well coordinated programme of activity for:

- improving the health of local people
- improving all the services having a bearing on people's health, whoever may provide them
- enabling all sections of the community to enjoy good health and access to services at need.

Each HImP covers a 3 year period. The first priority was to establish strong working partnerships. More comprehensive programmes will come into force after this. In preparing a programme, using processes already in hand and building on forward looking activities, account should be taken of:

- the government guidance on national priorities
- the public health White Paper *Our Healthier Nation*
- the White Papers *Modernising Social Services* and *Modern Local Government in Touch With the People*
- ways of using funds earmarked for NHS modernisation
- national service frameworks as they become available
- service and financial frameworks (SaFFs)
- national recommendations for organising services, e.g. The Calman-Hine Report for cancer services
- joint health and social services investment plans for older people.

## Health Professions Council see Council for Professions Supplementary to Medicine

## ⬚ Health Promotion Authority for Wales
The role of this body is to improve the health of the people of Wales to a level comparable to the best in Europe. Its work is based on partnerships and building health alliances across a range of groups and sectors. It is guided by The 'All in Wales' strategy. ✉

## ⬚ Health and Safety Commission
This Commission is responsible to the appropriate ministers for the administration of the Health and Safety at Work Act 1974. It is required to ensure that risks to people's health and safety from work activities are properly controlled. It reviews health and safety legislation and makes proposals for new or revised regulations and standards.

## ⬚ Health and Safety Executive
This is a body which advises and assists the Health and Safety Commission in its functions. The Executive has some specific statutory responsibilities including the enforcement of health

and safety law. The team includes a range of experts, including technologists, doctors, lawyers and scientists. ✉ ☾ ☞

## Health and Safety at Work Act 1974

The Health and Safety at Work Act is designed to provide the legislative framework to promote, stimulate and encourage high standards of health and safety at work. Part 1 of the Act relates to health, safety and welfare at work. It covers all 'persons at work' – employers, employees and the self-employed (apart from domestic servants in a private household), many of whom were not covered by previous legislation. It also covers the general public whose health may be affected by work activities. Employers must consider the specific issues associated with their area of work and the consequential training needs that arise for their organisations, such as lifting and handling in the health services. Since the loss of Crown Immunity in April 1991 for all NHS properties, these are now subject to the statutory requirements of the Health and Safety at Work Act. Thus all premises must abide by national fire regulation standards and observe the requirements of COSHH (control of substances hazardous to health) regulations and other related regulations.

## ▨ Health Service Commissioner (Ombudsman) see Complaints

Since 1997, the Health Service Commissioner (HSC) has been responsible for all complaints, including those in relation to clinical judgements. He or she cannot investigate areas relating to personnel or contractual matters, or where there has been recourse to a tribunal or the courts. The complaints will be investigated in full and a report sent to the complainant giving information on the investigations, the findings and any recommendations. Such recommendations are advisory, as the HSC does not have the power to require action of the Trust, health authority or GP. However, any failures to act on the recommendations are likely to be highlighted in the HSC's annual report, with a resultant invitation to explain the lack of action to the parliamentary select committee which reviews the work of the ombudsman. ✉ ☾ ☞

## ▨ Health and Social Services Executive, Northern Ireland

The Health and Social Services Executive (HSSE) manages health and social services in Northern Ireland. The Chief Executive works through individual directorates, such as Child and Community Care Directorate, Trust and Human Resources Directorate and Health Services Audit Directorate. Health is delivered through the four health and social services boards (HSSB).

## Healthcare professionals

The health services require a range of healthcare professionals each with their own unique role, although partnership working is becoming more and more common as cross-boundary activity is increasing. Roles and professional boundaries are coming under increasing scrutiny and some role experimentation, for example, between house officers and registered nurses, is taking place. Practitioners may work within the NHS, independent sector or privately, although this varies considerably from profession to profession. In essence, the core role of the individual professionals is as follows:

- *chiropodists*: see *podiatrists*
- *chiropractors*: treat disorders of the joints especially spinal injuries
- *clinical psychologists*: work with individuals or groups to explore, change or modify behaviour
- *dentists*: treat disorders of the teeth, mouth, gums, undertaking oral and maxillofacial and restorative surgery and orthodontics
- *dietitians*: apply the science of nutrition to the promotion of health and treatment of disease
- *dispensing opticians*: dispense and supply spectacles but must be specially certified to fit contact lenses
- *doctors*: diagnose and treat health problems through surgical or medical intervention
- *health visitors*: work as family visitors providing health education and social advice
- *medical laboratory science technicians*: carry out investigations to provide scientific evidence to support the clinical decision making of clinicians. Their major areas of specialisation are

H

clinical chemistry, haematology, blood transfusion, cellular pathology, medical microbiology and immunology

- *midwives*: work with women throughout all stages of pregnancy and childbirth to ensure optimum care for mother and baby. They manage the entire process of normal pregnancies
- *nurses*: give physical and psychological care to patients and clients, assisting them with the activities of daily living that they would undertake for themselves if well enough, and carrying out a range of nursing care and treatment
- *occupational therapists*: treat physical and mental health problems using specific activities. They work mainly with patients/clients who have problems as a result of physical disabilities, mental ill health or learning difficulties
- *optometrists*: test sight and prescribe and dispense spectacles and other optical appliances
- *orthoptists (also known as ophthalmic opticians)*: diagnose and treat defects of vision, eye position and abnormalities of eye movement
- *osteopaths*: treat disorders of the skeleton by manipulation and massage
- *pharmacists*: dispense medications and advice on the use and interaction of drugs
- *physiotherapists*: help to rehabilitate those who have suffered loss of physical function as a result of illness, old age or injury, such as sports injuries
- *podiatrists*: provide a comprehensive foot healthcare service
- *prosthetists and orthotists*: supply artificial limbs, other parts and mechanical aids
- *psychiatrists*: specialise, as doctors, in mental health problems
- *radiographers*: produce images utilising X-rays, radioisotopes, ultrasound and magnetic fields. Such images are used in the diagnosis and in monitoring the progress of disease.

In addition, there is also a range of smaller groups of administrative and technical staff who support the work of the health services. These include, for example, contact lens technicians, dental hygienists, medical photographers, phlebotomists and respiratory function technicians.

## Healthy living centres

Healthy living centres are national lottery funded facilities to help address the health and social needs of deprived communities. They can take a number of forms and offer a range of services such as food cooperatives, exercise classes and complementary therapies. They are likely to be housed in buildings but could also be virtual centres such as a healthy eating website. They are not a new idea but have been given impetus with National Lottery monies, with a total of £3 million being ring-fenced.

## Higher level practice

This describes the standard that the UKCC is proposing for those registered nurses working beyond the competencies associated with registration and experience. In due course, to be recognised by the UKCC as practising at a higher level, and to be registered accordingly, a nurse, midwife or health visitor would need to meet all the criteria in relation to:

- *providing effective health care*: e.g. 'receive direct referrals and undertake differential diagnosis using therapeutic communication, and valid, reliable and comprehensive patient and client centred assessments'
- *improving quality and health outcomes*: e.g. 'actively monitor the effectiveness of current therapeutic regimes and integrate practice to improve health outcomes in the interests of patients and clients'
- *evaluation and research*: e.g. 'critically appraise, synthesise and apply outcomes of relevant research, past evaluations and audits into practice to make improvements in the interests of patients and clients'
- *leading and developing practice*: e.g. 'working collaboratively and in partnership with other professionals'
- *innovation and changing practice*: e.g. 'develop appropriate strategies to make best use of resources in the interests of patients and clients and to achieve health outcomes'
- *developing self and others*: e.g. 'contribute to planning, developing and delivering learning and development opportunities for their own and other professions'

- *working across professional and organisational boundaries*:
  e.g. 'develop and apply strategies to learn effectively from
  others' knowledge and practice'.

Pilot schemes were undertaken in 2000 before a formal roll-
out of the scheme.

## Hospices

The concept of a hospice is that of a caring community – usually
run as a charity – of professional and non-professional people
together with the family. Emphasis is on dealing with the emotional and spiritual problems as well as the nursing and medical
problems of the terminally ill. Control of pain and other symptoms, keeping the patient at home for as long as possible or
desirable, and making the remaining days as comfortable as
possible are of primary concern. Relatives and carers are also
supported following bereavement.

## Human Rights Act 1998

The Human Right Act (HRA) which came into effect in October
2000 incorporates the European Convention on Human Rights
into domestic law. It will allow individuals to claim their rights
under the European Convention on Human Rights in UK courts
and tribunals instead of having to go to Strasbourg. It establishes, for example, the right to life, respect for private and family life, freedom from inhumane and degrading treatment and
freedom from arbitrary detention. Whilst, at the time of writing,
the full effect of the Act on all aspects of healthcare is unknown,
its implications could be considerable, particularly within the
field of mental health. Known as a 'higher law', successful challenges to it may result in the government being forced to change
aspects of domestic law to bring it into line with the principles of
human rights.

# A–Z guide

## ▧ Independent Healthcare Association

The Independent Healthcare Association (IHA) is the leading trade association of the UK's independent health and social care sector. Members include those who provide a range of services, such as nursing and residential care, elective surgery, psychiatric and substance abuse services and day surgery. The independent sector provides more health and social care beds (440 000) than the NHS and local authorities combined (356 000). ✉ ☎ 🗎 🖰

## Independent healthcare provision

Whilst the NHS remains the main provider of healthcare in the UK, an increasingly mixed economy in healthcare means that a growing number of individuals receive treatment within the independent (private) sector. The independent sector offers both acute and long-term care. It covers independent hospitals, both acute and mental health, substance abuse units, nursing and residential care homes, pathology laboratories, screening units, and day surgeries. Both commercial and charitable concerns offer a range of innovative and flexible services to those who need them. Employing over 449 000 people, the independent health and social care sector makes a significant contribution to the health of the nation. The largest growth area since the 1980s, representing a 25% increase, has been in the registered nursing residential and long stay homes and hospitals for the elderly, chronically sick and physically disabled.

## Information management

Information management is the term used to describe the process whereby information is 'managed' or used in such a way as to achieve the intended outcome. Information results from the processing of data – raw data in itself may not be helpful as it may not be in a format which is accessible or useable. Information may be managed via a number of communication processes or channels, i.e. line management structures, general meetings, notice boards, paper memoranda or by the use of information technology. The Government has taken the management of information very seriously, and in September 1998 published a White Paper entitled *Information for health. An Information Strategy for the Modern NHS 1998–2005* (NHSE 1998a).

## Inspection of nursing and residential homes

At the time of writing, the responsibility for inspection and regulation of nursing homes (including acute private hospitals) and residential homes lies with the health authorities and the social services respectively. Some homes have dual registration and thus must be inspected by both agencies. The Care Standards Bill was published by the Government in December 1999 and contains wide scale reforms of all inspection and regulation processes for homes for the elderly, the disabled and children. It will establish an independent National Care Standards Commission (NCSC) to regulate services for these groups, and will have the authority to close services down if appropriate. It will also have the responsibility of regulating private and voluntary hospitals and clinics. The intention is that the NCSC is active by Spring 2002.

## Institute of Health Service Managers
see **Institute of Healthcare Management**

## ▨ Institute of Healthcare Management

In 1999, the Institute of Health Service Managers (IHSM) joined with the Association of Managers in General Practice (AMGP) to form the new Institute of Healthcare Management to represent the interests of nearly 10000 healthcare managers. Its remit is to ensure that the managers' voice is heard and respected. It also devotes much of its time to ensuring that managers are equipped to handle the fast changing landscape of the NHS by actively promoting continuing professional development. Its membership, which is drawn from all sectors and sections of healthcare – from management trainees to chief executives, and everyone in between – is supported by the provision of a regional structure that arranges business and professional training.

# Intermediate care

Intermediate care is a broadly defined concept incorporating the care of patients who do not need acute tertiary care in hospitals but are not yet sufficiently independent to be self-caring within their own homes. The form intermediate care takes can vary but it is frequently offered in community hospitals and may be primarily nurse-led, with an emphasis on rehabilitation.

# International Council of Nurses

The International Council of Nurses (ICN) was established early this century, its first president being UK nurse Ethel Bedford Fenwick. It is the international forum for national nursing associations and its current membership stands at 118 countries. Its key role is to benchmark good nursing practice worldwide and to play a significant role in nursing education and in developing leadership programmes. It is also a seminal authority on nursing regulation. $\boxtimes$ ① 🖰

# International mobility of healthcare professionals

Healthcare professionals have traditionally been a fairly mobile group, often travelling to different countries to expand and enhance their professional experience or offering their services to developing countries. Requirements for travel and work in other countries vary considerably from place to place and should always be checked with the country concerned, either directly or through the relevant embassy in the UK. In many countries and in many professions a distinction will be made between relevant qualifications, registration and/or the licence to practise one's profession and employment requirements. These can be complex, time-consuming and expensive and ideally should be thoroughly researched before even considering travel.

## European Union

In theory, those individuals who are EU nationals and who qualify in an EU country have freedom of movement within the EU. In practice, this may mean that whilst registration or licence to practise in the host country is 'automatic' by means of the relevant EEC directive, there will frequently be local employment requirements which will delay or impede an individual's ability to actually practise their chosen profession. Individuals wishing to explore the requirements in further detail should contact either their professional organisation or their own registration body in the UK, who will be able to supply them with the relevant paperwork for application to the host competent or designated authority.

*Competent authority* is the body dealing with the professions with sectoral, or profession-specific directives. In health, these are: dentists, doctors, midwives, nurses responsible for general care, pharmacists, GPs and veterinary surgeons.

*Designated authority* is the body dealing with the professions who do not have profession-specific directives, such as the professions supplementary to medicine.

### Movement outside the EU

There is no general freedom of movement outside the EU although for some healthcare professions many countries have reciprocal arrangements with others. In each case, the interested individual should check the specific requirements with the host country.

### Incoming migrants

Healthcare professionals who have qualified outside the UK and who wish to work in the UK should check the requirements for registration/licence to practise and for employment before entering the UK. The bodies concerned have different responsibilities for different aspects of the process. For example, the relevant profession-specific statutory body, such as the UKCC or GMC, will consider applications for UK registration from nurses/midwives and doctors respectively, without which practice is not legal in the UK. The Home Office will deal with work permits. Professional organisations may be able to give advice on employment possibilities. The fragmentation of roles and responsibilities can make the process of registration and employment a frustrating, tortuous and expensive business for many incoming applicants.

# A–Z guide

## King's Fund

The King's Fund is a charity founded over 100 years ago by King Edward VII. Prior to the formation of the NHS, the money from the charity went to help run London's hospitals. It carries out research and development work, to bring about better health policies and services. Its main focus of work is London but it also works nationally and internationally.

The King's Fund is seen as an independent voice in health. Its key goals are:

- to reduce inequalities in health
- to promote cultural diversity
- to encourage joint working between professionals and organisations responsible for health and social care, and
- to involve the public in making decisions about health.

The Fund gives particular attention to groups of people who experience social exclusion such as older people, minority ethnic groups, people with mental health problems, carers and refugees. The King's Fund works across a broad spectrum of health issues to achieve its key goals. It concentrates on areas where the need is greatest:

- *Community care*: Working to improve and integrate services for people with long-term health and social care needs, in particular vulnerable older people and those with mental health problems.
- *Effective practice*: Working with health professionals to develop care that is effective, efficient and responsive to patient's needs. It is looking at the new system for clinical governance and the NHS and the ways the different professions are regulated.
- *Health systems*: Developing an overview of the systems that underlie health and social care, monitoring how London's

health services are funded and provided and comparing them against national and international standards.

- *Primary care*: Working to improve the quality of primary care. Projects include evaluating new ways of providing primary care and helping the new primary care groups as they take over responsibility for commissioning and providing health services.
- *Public health*: Exploring new ways to tackle the wide inequalities in society that have an effect on people's health. Work includes an evaluation of ways in which communities can be involved in efforts to make their local environments more healthy, and an examination of the likely impact of the Greater London Authority on people's health.
- *Living values*: Working to stimulate public debate on the values which underpin the NHS. Hopefully this will bring people from all backgrounds together to talk about their priorities for health and social care and to become more closely involved in public policy debate.

The King's Fund organises conferences and seminars with the intent of influencing policy development at government level and maintains close links to health services by established management development programmes for managers, clinicians and chairmen.

## A–Z guide

## Leadership and management in healthcare

Often, the terms leadership and management are confused, and used interchangeably. Simply put, *leadership* entails inspiring and motivating people to achieve. It is about innovation and creativity. *Management*, however, is more about process and systems, and the ability to achieve the task against a set of benchmarks. Neither quality is mutually exclusive. Some people are good leaders, but weak managers, some are good managers, but lack leadership ability. Some people can do both, either simultaneously or at different times in different contexts.

The important thing is that we need both contributions: healthcare needs good leadership and good management. However, whilst usually most leadership is seen as being a good thing, in that it takes the service forward, management and managers are not always given the same support. However, one cannot be effective without the other, and thus we should value both attributes equally. Innovative leadership, spearheading new ways of thinking, needs effective management to see through the ideas, and to ensure that robust systems are there to protect the public and the organisation.

## Legal aspects of healthcare

### Fulfilling expectations

Broadly speaking, UK legislation does provide a general right to healthcare. The National Health Service Act 1977 guarantees anyone the right to a local surgery for routine treatment as well as placing GPs under a duty to act in any emergency within their area. However, whilst hospitals must respond in similarly urgent cases, hospital admissions have depended upon practical considerations such as facilities and funding rather than absolute right.

## Reaching agreement and sharing responsibilities

Any relationship between the healthcare professional and the patient is centred on consent, competence and confidentiality. No treatment can be legally administered without permission. Intentional physical contact with others in an aggressive, offensive or invasive manner without their consent constitutes a trespass to the person. From informal examination to major surgery, the courts have emphasised that mutual communication between healthcare staff and patients is needed to ensure that such consent is properly obtained. All patients have the right to expect competent advice and treatment. Clearly, whilst the onus is on the healthcare professional's duty to safeguard this standard of care regardless, it is only common sense that patients who cooperate in their treatment help themselves as well. Strictly speaking, all healthcare professionals must respect the confidence of their patients and a successful relationship will often depend on such confidentiality. Breaches of patient confidence are, on the whole, rare but have been justified commonly on the basis of the patient's own welfare or the public interest. Healthcare staff are expected to be as open and honest with their patients as is reasonable but mutual trust can develop only if the patients themselves respond in the same way. Here again, the more responsible patients are towards their own treatment the more effective it can be.

## Counting the cost

Ultimately, however, the responsibility for a patient's healthcare lies with the medical professions. Acts of trespass, negligence or breaches of confidentiality have generated a variety of claims for compensation made by patients against those involved. In its broadest sense, legal liability is collective. Whilst individual professionals employed by a surgery or hospital are professionally accountable for their mistakes, it will be the GP who employs them or the local health authority recognised in law as being vicariously responsible for their employees' conduct that is generally the body who bears the cost. Nevertheless, malpractice litigation is expensive and for relatively minor grievances, it will be more appropriate to rely on the formal complaints procedure available. Both the work of the Health Service Commissioner and the wide disciplinary powers of the statutory bodies such as the GMC and the UKCC reinforce the patients' right of redress.

## Establishing safeguards

The health and safety of the patient, which is safeguarded both by common law and by public liability legislation, is extended by the Health and Safety at Work Act 1974 to protecting staff at work against general and specific risks. Both surgeries and hospitals are required by law to reinforce rigorous health and safety policies covering the standards of the premises as well as the conduct of the staff themselves. The handling of equipment, samples and substances is just one of the many health and safety aspects to be considered.

## Reviewing boundaries

Medical law is a balance between the practical and the permissible. Reluctance to find fault with healthcare professionals, especially doctors, is based on the maintenance of public confidence. This must, however, be set against the patient's inalienable right to expect that his or her physical and mental wellbeing is being respected by those who often have that person's life in their hands. Responsible healthcare depends upon mutual cooperation between patient and healthcare professional within the boundaries set by law.

# Legislative process of a government bill

The process for making law in the UK parliament depends upon the type of legislation concerned. All Acts will begin life as a bill. Draftsmen compose the bill and the end product is presented to the House of Commons.

## First reading

The clerk to the House will read the short title of the bill and the relevant minister, or his or her representative, will name a day for the second reading.

## Statement of compatibility

Before the second reading, the minister in charge of a bill must make a statement of compatibility in relation to the European Convention of Human Rights (s19 Human Rights Act 1998). Alternatively, the statement must indicate that whilst this is not possible, the Government wishes to proceed with the bill.

### Second reading

The House will consider and debate the principles behind the bill. Second readings can be refused, though this is rare. Non-controversial bills can be dealt with in a second reading committee.

### Money resolutions and ways and means resolutions

It is normal for these to be dealt with after the second reading and before the committee stage. Money resolutions authorise those parts of a bill which will drain significant sums from central government funds. To authorise the levying of taxes and other charges, ways and means resolutions are required.

### Committee stage

The bill is examined clause by clause. The committee may make amendments and introduce new clauses within the limits of the subject matter. Routine bills will generally go to a standing committee – that is, a group of members reflecting the party divide of the House. The whole House may consider a bill at committee stage. This generally happens with bills of constitutional importance.

### Report stage

The bill is reviewed in light of amendments made during the committee stage. Further amendments may be made and all members can speak and vote. Where a bill has been dealt with by a committee of the whole House, and no amendments are made, there will be no report stage.

### Third reading

The House will review the bill, given the amendments made at committee and report stage. There can be no substantive amendments made during this stage.

### House of Lords

The bill will now be sent to the House of Lords where the legislative process is currently basically the same as in the Commons. One noticeable difference is that bills are usually considered in a committee of the whole House. Both the Lords and the Commons must agree the final text of the bill. Where there is conflict, the Parliament Act 1949 provides that the Commons will prevail.

### Royal assent

The Crown is the third element in the composition of Parliament. Before a bill can become law, it requires royal assent.

### Commencement orders

Not all Acts come into force on the date of royal assent. A commencement order may be used to bring some or all of the provisions of an Act into force. A commencement order is a form of secondary legislation.

### Hansard

Debate in each House is reported in Hansard and the text can be invaluable in understanding the intention of Parliament when construing an Act.

### Amendment

Historically, amendment of primary legislation has been by further primary legislation. Increasingly, however, amendments may be effected by secondary legislation (statutory instruments) which can be introduced on the direction of a minister and which can be the subject of approval merely by means of being laid before the House of Commons. This power is derived from what are known as *Henry VIII clauses*, which Henry VIII introduced at a time when he could not be certain that Parliament would authorise his matrimonial wishes.

## Lifelong learning

The concept of lifelong learning has gradually gained momentum since the mid-1980s. There are a number of terms that are used interchangeably – continuous development, continuous learning, permanent education, self-directed learning – but lifelong learning is the most commonly used. The European Year of Lifelong Learning was in 1996, demonstrating a wider recognition that the demands of a society which is constantly changing require rapidly changing skills on the part of those who wish to work within it. It is linked with continuing professional development and portfolio careers.

A number of trends have been identified in relation to lifelong learning (Wallace 1999), including:

- an expansion of educational services outside the 'normal' school age – both before the conventional start of education and after it has finished
- an awareness, acceptance and embracing of the idea that 'learning' does not stop at the end of formal or statutory education
- a greater interest in education and learning as a means of improving the quality of life
- an enhanced awareness of the relevance and applicability of education to the demands of day-to-day life, rather than as a separate entity
- an increased realisation that specific job skills have a tendency to become obsolete very quickly
- a greater participation in decisions about education by a greater number of people, including parents, members of the public and consumers of education – both adults and children.

Such an approach is highly relevant to those working in healthcare as they strive to keep their knowledge and skills up-to-date in a rapidly changing environment.

## Living Wills see Advance Directives

## Local health councils, Scotland see Community Health Councils

## Local health groups see Primary Care Groups

## ▨ Long-term Medical Conditions Alliance

The Long-term Medical Conditions Alliance (LMCA) is the umbrella body for national voluntary organisations working to meet the needs of people with long-term conditions. Over 700 000 people belong to its 110 member organisations. It aims to ensure that the voice of people with long-term illness is heard and it provides support to its members. ✉ ① 📄 @ ⌐

## Managed care

A system of care originally used in the USA by managed care companies who provide guidelines for the care and treatment of each patient. Healthcare practitioners have had concerns for several years that this system does not deliver quality care, with patients being denied cover, particularly in relation to prescription drugs and health plan decisions, resulting in a decline in health for the patients concerned. Practitioners are expected to adhere to the guidelines or risk losing the business. The system is justified on the basis that:

- it is a means of controlling inflationary health costs
- the therapeutic relationship is subjected to scrutiny and evaluation
- it increases the accountability of clinicians
- it increases client involvement and client responsibility for care and treatment
- it promotes cost-effective and short-term inventions
- it requires realistic therapeutic goals
- it promotes outcome research.

## Managed Clinical Networks

Managed Clinical Networks (MCNs) are defined as 'linked groups of health professionals and organisations from primary, secondary and tertiary care, working in a co-ordinated way, unconstrained by existing professional and Health Board boundaries, to ensure equitable provision of high quality clinically effective services throughout Scotland' (Scottish Executive NHS MEL 1999).

The networks, which must be agreed and approved, must be governed by the following core principles:

- managed not drifting, so that there are clear structures and lines of responsibility; one person taking overall responsibility but clear roles for all

- purpose is to improve patient care in terms of quality of care, access, convenience and coordination of care
- work undertaken must be evidence based using SIGN guidelines and protocols where appropriate; networks will support research and development
- outcomes need to be measured and audit will be an integral part of the work
- a quality assurance programme will be required which is acceptable to the Clinical Standards Board for Scotland
- each network will produce a written annual report, which will be available to the public
- must be truly multidisciplinary and multiprofessional; all the disciplines involved must be valued as clinicians in their own right; need appropriately trained clinicians working in partnership with adequate facilities
- patients must be involved in shaping the network and each network will have a policy on disseminating information.

##  Medical Defence Union

The Medical Defence Union (MDU) was founded in 1885 originally by doctors, for doctors. It is a mutual, non-profit-making organisation owned by its membership of doctors, dentists, nurses and other healthcare professionals. It defends the professional reputation of its members when their skills are called into question. On their behalf, it pays legal costs in the civil courts and pays damages to patients who have suffered as a result of a medical mishap during treatment. It provides a range of professional information and educational material. ✉ ☏ 📄 @

## Medical Royal Colleges

The Medical Royal Colleges are professional associations of medical practitioners covering a wide range of medical specialties. They are all broadly responsible for setting education standards within their own specialty and undertake a varying range of education and training activities. The ones detailed below are for illustrative purposes only. Names and contact details of all the colleges are contained in Appendix 1 at the end of the book.

The **Royal College of Physicians of Edinburgh** was formed in 1681 with the purpose of advancing medicine as a reputable science and alleviating the miseries of the city's poor and needy. It currently works to promote the highest standards of internal medicine, not only in Edinburgh but worldwide. The college acts in an advisory capacity to government and other organisations and has a strong commitment to audit and research. It organises a range of professional development activities for doctors and other healthcare professionals. ✉ ① 📄

🕿 The **Royal College of Surgeons of England** undertakes a wide range of activities, including: the supervision of training posts, courses and workshops for surgeons and others, examinations, the promotion of research, collaboration with other national and international bodies, and as an advisory body to a range of governmental and other organisations. ✉ ① ☝

🕿 The **Royal College of Paediatrics and Child Health** is one of the newer royal colleges. The British Paediatric Association was granted royal college status in 1996. Its main functions are to advance the art and science of paediatrics, to improve standards of medical care to children and to educate and examine doctors in paediatrics.

🕿 The **Royal College of General Practitioners (RCGP)** exists to encourage, foster and maintain the highest possible standards in general medical practice. ✉ ① 📄 ☝

## 🕿 Medicines Control Agency

The Medicines Control Agency (MCA) is an executive agency of the Department of Health. Its main function is to safeguard public health by ensuring that all medicines – both branded and non-branded – on the UK market meet acceptable standards of safety, quality and efficacy.

Medicines which reach the standard are granted a marketing authorisation, which used to be known as a product licence. Those products which have been granted such authorisation carry a number prefixed with PL on the pack. There are three categories for the supply of medicines:

- *General sales list (GSL) medicines*, which are widely available for sale and use without supervision of a pharmacist or doctor
- *Pharmacy (P) medicines*, which can only be obtained from a pharmacy, where they are supplied under the supervision of the pharmacist, who may check whether the medicine is necessary and the one most appropriate to meet a person's needs

- *Prescription only medicines (POM)*, which must be prescribed by a doctor or dentist. They can be obtained from a pharmacy.

✉ ☽ 🗎

## ▨ Mental Health Act Commission ✉
see **Mental Welfare Commission**

## Mental health national service framework
see **National service frameworks**

## ▨ Mental Welfare Commission

There are two commissions within the UK, each established to provide specific functions with regard to individuals with mental health problems. The Mental Welfare Commission was established within Scotland and the Mental Health Act Commission within England. Although the English Commission is purely concerned with detained patients, the following is a brief overview of both.

The 1984 Mental Health Act (Scotland) called for the Mental Health Commission to be established and requires it to have a minimum of 10 commissioners, of whom at least 3 must be women, 3 must be medical commissioners and 1 must be a lawyer. The Commission is widely held to be a guardian of the interests of individual patients and has powers of release of detained patients (i.e. those held under the Act). It acts in place of the NHS ombudsman in the NHS complaints procedures for patients with mental disorders and visits every psychiatric and learning disability hospital at least once a year. It publishes an annual report and in other ways seeks to promote good practice in the operation of the Act. A major part of the Commission's work is to conduct enquiries into cases of apparent deficiency in care. The Commission is in many ways a unique body but it may be possible to compare its powers and roles with those of other bodies, such as the Equal Opportunities Commission, which have responsibilities both to assist and to promote the general principles of their founding legislation. ✉ ☽

## Mentoring

Mentoring in the traditional sense involves a confidential relationship between one person who is more experienced – usually more senior – and one who is less experienced – the protégé or mentee. The mentor offers advice and support while the overall purpose is to promote learning and development.

The process is characterised by sharing of experience, problem solving and coaching. The origin of this traditional approach is found in the concept of apprenticeship, associated with master craftsmen, sports coaches and athletes. The name originally came from the local wise man, called Mentor, with whom Odysseus left his son when setting off on his legendary journeys. It soon passed into the language as a synonym for a wise and trusted advisor. Within a large organisation, mentorship will go beyond teaching, instruction and passing on practical skills. It will involve career advice, life planning and networking. According to Clutterbuck (1997) the mentor becomes interested in the protégé's personal development and lifelong learning.

Mentors will look out for the individual interests of their mentees, be on their side and guide them in accessing important networks. The mentor will also act as a role model. However, Hay (1997) argues that as organisations become flatter in structure and leaner in the number of middle management positions, the traditional approach to mentoring is no longer relevant. The traditional 'old boy' network is discriminatory and cloning managers is an inappropriate approach to fast changing environments. Hay also suggests that there are insufficient numbers of senior people within organisations to sustain the mentoring role. A new approach is called for, referred to by Hay (1997) as a 'developmental alliance'. This new approach is characterised by a relationship between equals. One or more of those involved will enable individuals to increase awareness of self and identify alternative strategies to take action to develop themselves. Mentors will set aside their own view of the world and be prepared to experiment with ideas and new ways of doing things.

Mentors in the traditional model were selected for their track record of success and the mentee was encouraged to follow them. Mentors in the developmental alliance model will need an understanding of the process of learning, which is different from teaching and coaching. It is about accessing deeper levels of awareness and the mentor and mentee play an equal part in that transformational process.

**M**

When choosing a mentor, the key elements to look for in the developmental alliance model are trust, respect and a shared ethical base. Mentees need to be able to reveal honestly and frankly their concerns about abilities and relationships. The choice of the mentor will be based less on the position of the individual in an organisation and more on his or her track record as an effective mentor.

## Midwifery

The role of the midwife is to 'be with' women, not to do for or to them, although this may be part of 'being with'. This can be difficult to define or recognise but is the foundation on which midwifery is based. Midwives are accountable for their practice in whatever environment they practise. They are responsible for providing care to mothers and babies in accordance with the *Midwives Code of Practice* (UKCC 1998a). The care covers prenatal, intranatal and postnatal periods and is designed to meet the needs of the individual woman and her child.

Care may be provided in the woman's home, at a health centre, GP's surgery or maternity hospital and the aim is to maintain and improve the standard of health of the woman concerned. Midwives provide advice on matters relating to pregnancy and health during that time and enable women to make informed choices. The European Community Directive 80/155/EEC Article 4 defines the activities of a midwife and specifies 'midwives are at least entitled to take up and pursue the following activities', which include:

- the provision of sound family planning advice
- diagnosis of pregnancy
- provision of prenatal care and parenthood classes
- education and care in labour
- conduct of deliveries
- recognition of abnormality in mother or baby
- care of both mother and child in the postnatal period.

As midwives are members of a multiprofessional group, these activities are not pursued in isolation and midwives work with doctors, health visitors and other professionals to provide high standards of care. Midwives also work with consumer associations, and the agenda for change in practice may be initiated by consumers, for example, increased requests for water births and non-intervention in labour.

## MIND

Established in 1946, MIND is the leading mental health charity in England and Wales. It works for a better life for people diagnosed or treated as mentally ill. It does this through campaigning, community development, training and publishing a comprehensive information service. MIND draws on the expertise of people with direct experience as providers and users of mental health services. Local MIND associations offer a range of services around the country including supported housing, crisis helplines, drop-in centres, befriending, advocacy, employment and training schemes. ✉ ☎ @ ⌐

## Manufacturing Science and Finance

Manufacturing Science and Finance (MSF) is a major trades union representing skilled and professional people in both the public and private sectors. Within the health services, its members include doctors, health visitors, pharmacists, scientific staff and speech therapists. ✉ ⌐

**M**

### ▓ National Association of Patient Participation

A voluntary network of patient groups working with GPs, primary care groups and Trusts. It has over 200 affiliated patient groups aiming to ensure that patients are able to represent their views and concerns. ✉ ☺

### ▓ National Audit Office

The Comptroller and Auditor General is responsible for examining accounts of government departments, certain public bodies and international organisations. The Comptroller reports to Parliament on the economy, efficiency and effectiveness of public spending. ✉ ☺ 📄

### ▓ National Back Pain Association ✉ ☺ ⌐ see BackCare

### ▓ National Board for Nursing, Midwifery and Health Visiting for Northern Ireland

The National Board for Nursing, Midwifery and Health Visiting for Northern Ireland (NBNI) was set up as a result of the Nurses, Midwives and Health Visitors Act 1979 and came into being on 1 July 1983. It was reconstituted as an executive non-departmental public body following the Nurses, Midwives and Health Visitors Act 1992, which was subsequently amended by the Nurses, Midwives and Health Visitors Act 1997. Its functions are to ensure that education and training for nurses, midwives and health visitors adhere to standards set by the UKCC. It also plays a key role in the strategic development of education and training for the professions, working closely with the Department of Health and Social Services, the UKCC, the other national boards and other healthcare agencies.

The current board consists of 7 non-executive members (including the Chair) and 2 executive members. Following a government review in 1998, the four national boards and the UKCC are to be replaced in 2001 by a UK central body to be known as the Nurses and Midwives Council. Arrangements for Northern Ireland were under consideration at the time of writing. (See also ENB, NBS, UKCC, WNB.) ✉ ☽ 🗎

## ▧ National Board for Nursing, Midwifery and Health Visiting for Scotland

The core business of the National Board for Nursing, Midwifery and Health Visiting for Scotland (NBS) is to ensure that the educational standards set by the UKCC are met in Scotland. Its central business is its research and development function which facilitates the assessment of the effectiveness and efficiency of the regulatory process and evaluates educational provision for nurses, midwives and health visitors. The NBS believes that sound evidence should underpin education and professional regulation. The NBS currently has 10 members, 3 executive and 7 non-executive. Following a government review in 1998, the four national boards and the UKCC are to be replaced by a new UK statutory body to be called the Nurses and Midwives Council. The nature of the four country representation is currently under consideration. Consultations are currently taking place regarding the nature, role and function of the body to succeed the NBS – probably to be called the Scottish Nursing and Midwifery Education Council. ✉ ☽ 🗎

## National confidential enquiries

The national confidential enquiries have been established over a period of several years to examine clinical performance and serious avoidable events. The results of the enquiries now form a key part of the data to be considered by the quality bodies, such as NICE. Relevant clinicians have a legal duty to participate in the enquiries. The four enquiries are:

- *National confidential enquiry into perioperative deaths (NCEPOD)*: established to encourage high standards of surgery and anaesthesia by auditing hospital deaths occurring within 30 days of any surgical or gynaecological operation.

- *Confidential enquiry into stillbirths and deaths in infancy (CESDI)*: established to identify ways to prevent stillbirths and infant deaths, including gaps in research.
- *Confidential enquiry into maternal deaths (CEMD)*: established to assess the main causes of and trends in maternal deaths, including gaps in research.
- *Confidential enquiry into suicide and homicide by people with mental illness (CISH)*: established to perform a national audit of suicide and homicide by people with a history of mental illness.

## National Council for Hospice and Specialist Palliative Care Services

The National Council for Hospice and Specialist Palliative Care Services provides information and services for all those concerned with the provision of hospice and specialist palliative care services. ✉ ☽ 🖹 @ ☝

## National Electronic Library for Health

The National Electronic Library for Health (NeLH [sic], http://www.nelh.nhs.uk/) is being developed to provide healthcare professionals and the general public with high quality health information. The NeLH is to be fully operational by March 2002 to 'provide easy access to best current knowledge and know-how' and 'improve health and healthcare, clinical practice and patient choice'. It is available via NHSnet and the Internet.

## National Information Forum

The National Information Forum (NIF) is concerned to ensure by all means possible that disabled people get the information they need to lead lives of choice in our communities. It has various publications which cover their interests, for example, *Disability Information in Hospitals, Signposts* (a guide to the key sources of information for disabled people), and *Innovations in Information*. It is also looking at information available on services in the community for asylum seekers and refugees. ✉ ☽ 🖹 ☝

## National information strategy

The NHS Executive published the new strategy for information in the NHS in September 1998. Local implementation strategies have to be developed which:

- articulate the links to the local HImPs, underpinning plans such as primary care investment and human resources
- recognise that information underpins the delivery of quality services as outlined in *A First Class Service* (DOH 1998a) and will support clinical governance plans
- support behavioural and cultural change from the use of information, and appropriate education, training and development programmes
- recognise that a strategy is dynamic and needs monitoring, reviewing and reassessing to ensure it keeps pace with technological change and new requirements.

## National Institute of Clinical Effectiveness

Introduced as part of the Government's clinical governance initiative in the White Paper *The New NHS: Modern, Dependable* (DOH 1997), the National Institute of Clinical Effectiveness (NICE) is an English special health authority. It is managed by a director and a small executive. The board of eight members consists of key health service professionals and lay representation.

It has a range of objectives:

- to produce clinical guidelines based on relevant evidence of clinical cost-effectiveness
- to introduce and disseminate associated clinical audit methodologies and information on good practice and clinical audit
- to bring together work currently being undertaken by the many professional organisations in receipt of Department of Health funding for this purpose
- to work with a programme agreed with and funded from current resources by the Department of Health.

A standard strategy is being used for each area under investigation, as follows:

- identifying and examining medicines and procedures that are likely to have a significant impact on the NHS
- examining current practices to identify unjustified variations in use or uncertainty about clinical or cost effectiveness of the intervention

**N**

- collecting evidence and undertaking research to assess the clinical and cost effectiveness of healthcare interventions
- considering the implications for clinical practice of the evidence on clinical and cost effectiveness and producing guidelines for the NHS
- dissemination of the guidance and supporting audit methodologies
- implementation at local level, through clinical governance and other approaches
- monitoring the impact of advice, taking into account the views of patients and their representatives and any relevant new research findings.

## National Plan

The National Plan was launched by the Secretary of State for Health in England in August 2000. Following an extensive public consultation process, the plan contains radical proposals for the future of the NHS. It covers a wide range of issues, including proposals for, amongst other things: increased consumer involvement, a mandatory reporting system for adverse incidents, increased information on health services, expansion and realignment of professional roles, changes to the current working patterns of NHS staff, such as medical consultants, the further development of NHS Direct online, greater lay membership of the regulatory bodies, and a UK Council of Health Regulators linking the numerous health regulatory bodies. National plans are also anticipated in Northern Ireland, Scotland and Wales.

## National register for carers

This is a voluntary register of carers, set up as an individual initiative by an interested individual in Liverpool in 1991. The register has over 32 000 members who are employed as carers. Checks are made on applicants and some are refused registration. The register has review procedures and a probationary scheme for the less experienced carers, or where doubts have been raised. The information on the register is available to employers.

## National schedule of reference costs

NHS Trusts will be required to publish their costs on a consistent basis and the data will be published in a national schedule of reference costs so that performance on efficiency can be benchmarked.

## National Schizophrenia Fellowship

The National Schizophrenia Fellowship (NSF) is the largest mental health charity in Europe. It exists to improve the lives of everyone affected by severe mental illnesses by providing quality support and services and by influencing local, regional and national policies. The NSF also provides information on the following:

- diagnosis and treatment of mental illness
- accommodation issues and respite care
- the rights of patients and relatives
- hospital admission and treatment
- community care and support
- legal matters
- rehabilitation and employment
- medication and complementary therapies
- benefits, grants and insurance.

## National service frameworks

National service frameworks (NSFs) will bring together the best evidence of clinical and cost effectiveness with the views of service users to determine the best ways of providing particular patient and care services. The intention is to reduce the 'postcode lottery' of available care and treatment by setting benchmarks and targets for the care and treatment of specific areas of practice. Mental health, coronary heart disease, older people and diabetes are all subjects which have been identified for national service frameworks.

The first national service framework was produced in 1999 in mental health and requires that all mental health services should:

- promote mental health for all and combat discrimination against people with mental health problems
- identify patients' needs and ensure they are offered effective treatments
- ensure all services are available round the clock
- ensure that all mental health service users on the care programme approach receive care that prevents or anticipates crisis and reduces risk

**N**

- provide a hospital bed or suitable alternative for those who need it, close to home
- make sure that carers have their needs assessed every year
- reduce suicide rates.

## Networking

Networking is an essential skill for all healthcare professionals. The pace of professional lives has made it the new and essential way of working. Although we know more than ever before, there is a need both to negotiate the complexities of organisational life and to self-manage our own professional development and career. Networking is active and dynamic and primarily about relationships. It is more than merely belonging to a network of like-minded people or those with a common interest, such as a professional organisation. The term originated from computer language used to describe a system of interconnected terminals and peripheral equipment in which each user has some access to others using the system whilst sharing internal and external memories and other capabilities. This analogy still has some legitimacy, although human networking has a greater flexibility and the capacity to be modified according to the needs of the participants. Networking is an ideal vehicle for sharing innovations with colleagues, dissemination of information about practice developments, formal recognition of good work, the cross fertilisation of ideas and the sharing of information.

## Neurological Alliance

The Neurological Alliance brings together individual neurological charities to pursue the highest standards of service and care for people affected by a neurological condition.

## NHS confederation

The NHS confederation was established in 1997 to represent the interests of all NHS bodies across the UK. Two former organisations, the Trust Federation and the National Association of Health Authorities and Trusts (NAHAT) merged to join the NHS confederation. Its principal concern is to promote the NHS to policy and decision makers, the media and the wider health community.

The confederation aims to influence policy and decision makers, the media and the wider health community by:

- providing a single credible reference point for expert comments on health and health service issues
- providing a range of opportunities for members' voices to be heard
- bringing people and organisations in the wider health community together to work in partnership in the interests of better health and healthcare
- building wider awareness and understanding of key health and health services issues via the media and other settings.

Policy work is overseen by a range of contributors and advisory groups. They deal with key areas including human resources, public health, learning disabilities, mental health, specialist Trusts, primary care and NHS resources. Working groups are established to tackle specific issues such as preparing evidence for enquiries or responding to consultation papers.

The organisation represents over 95% of all statutory NHS management bodies across the UK, e.g. NHS Trusts, health authorities and health boards. Some GP commissioning bodies are also affiliated. Associate status is available to CHCs and local health councils, national organisations concerned with health, academic departments, non-NHS statutory agencies, independent healthcare companies and bodies, and their associations. The confederation is an independent charity. It is managed by a board of trustees which is drawn from the elected councils, one comprising representatives of member health authorities and the other of NHS Trusts. The councils, which always meet together, are responsible for key policy and representational issues. Council membership is comprised of members from the regions and territories and it acts as the lynch-pin within the broader membership. The confederation operates a regional structure in England which mirrors the NHS Executive regions. This provides opportunities to network with members and partners. It is a strong intelligence network and the basis for a database of experts. Wales has its own confederation branch, which provides excellent opportunities to network with members and partners in the Principality. The intention is to set up similar bodies in Scotland and Northern Ireland to reflect the distinctive nature of the NHS in each of these countries.

**N**

## ▨ NHS Direct

Proposed in the White Paper *The New NHS: Modern, Dependable* (DOH 1997), NHS Direct is an initiative which started in 1998 to provide a 24-hour confidential helpline staffed by registered nurses and trained operators in England. It is gradually being rolled out across the UK. Nurses use accredited clinical guidelines, with accompanying computer software, prompting them on the appropriate questions to ask and on advice to give callers. Where appropriate, advice on self-care is given, a referral to a GP suggested or arranged, or an ambulance called.

The objectives of the service are to:

- offer the public confidential, reliable and consistent source of professional advice on healthcare 24 hours a day, so that they can manage many of their problems at home or know where to turn for the appropriate care
- provide simple and speedy access to a comprehensive and up-to-date range of health and related information
- help improve quality, increase cost-effectiveness and reduce unnecessary demands on other NHS services by providing a more appropriate response to the needs of the public
- allow professionals to develop their role in enabling patients to be partners in self-care and help them focus on those patients for whom their skills are most needed.

It is designed to give immediate information and friendly advice on worrying health problems – on what to do, or not to do – at any time of day or night. It is designed for those who are not sure whether to call out their doctor or go to accident and emergency departments. It provides people at home with easier and faster advice about health, illness and the NHS so that they are better able to care for themselves and their families. Implemented initially in a limited number of pilot sites, the government commitment is for full national roll-out by the end of 2000. Despite reservations expressed by some GPs, early evaluations show very positive responses from the public. A formal evaluation of the first wave of pilot sites is being undertaken by the Medical Research Unit at Sheffield University.
◑ ✍

## ▧ NHS Direct online

NHS Direct online offers finger tip access to an interactive self-care guide based on the top 20 symptoms on which callers most frequently seek advice from the telephone helpline. It will also provide accredited information about hundreds of diseases and self-care groups. It can be found at www. nhsdirect.nhs.uk.

## ▧ NHS Information Management and Technology electronic library

The NHS Information Management and Technology (IM&T) electronic library is an online information service for those involved in the management and delivery of IM&T within the English Health Service. For more information go to http://www. ctf.imc.exec.nhs.uk/.

## ▧ NHS Information Authority

The NHS Information Authority was set up as a special health authority in April 1999. Its responsibilities include developing national products and standards to support local implementation of the new information strategy and ensuring that the NHS has high quality information to support the core functions of the NHS in caring for individuals and improving public health. It will work in partnership with a range of individuals and bodies with an interest in the NHS.

## NHS net

This is intended to be an internal electronic superhighway for the NHS, scheduled to take effect from 2005. It will be used, for example, for:

- the transfer of patient information, including between general practice and hospitals, available 24 hours a day
- a discussion forum
- diagnostic support
- evidence-based practice
- electronic books
- video training banks.

It will be designed as an 'intranet', that is an electronic net to give users the power to access all the information that they need within a controlled environment of private networks to protect security and confidentiality.

## NHS Pension Scheme

The NHS Pension Scheme (the Scheme) is a statutory scheme administered by the NHS Pensions Agency, which is an executive agency of the Department of Health. Contributions from both members and employers are paid to the Exchequer, which meet the costs of the Scheme benefits. The rules of the Scheme are laid down in the 1995 NHS Pension Scheme Regulations. The Scheme is an extremely valuable benefit for people working in the NHS, not least because the package of benefits is fully protected against inflation and is guaranteed by the Government. Membership of the Scheme is open to any NHS employee aged between 16 and 70 and all NHS medical, dental and ophthalmic practitioners, including trainees, some locums and assistants. Some members of the Scheme who leave the NHS to work for approved organisations outside the NHS, for example, hospices, are also entitled to remain as members.

The Scheme provides:

- a retirement pension based on 1/80th of an employee's pay at retirement for each year of the Scheme membership. This scheme is therefore what is known as a 'final salary' scheme and not a 'money purchase' scheme, which is the norm for private pensions. The latter is more risky since it is based upon the value of stocks and shares, at the date of retire-ment, which have been purchased by the pension contributions
- a tax free lump sum on retirement equal to three times the employee's pension
- life assurance payment equivalent to 2 years' pay if the employee dies before he or she retires. Payment and allowances for an employee's spouse and children on the employee's death
- benefits if the employee has to retire because of ill-health after 2 years' membership and enhanced benefits after 5 years' membership. If an employee is seriously ill and does not expect to live longer than 1 year, he or she can apply for a larger lump sum instead of a pension

- improved benefits if an employee is made redundant at or after the age of 50 and has at least 5 years of membership.

### Retirement age

The normal retirement age for most Scheme members is 60. An employee is entitled to take voluntary early retirement on or after the age of 50. However, benefits will be reduced to cover the extra costs of receiving a pension for a longer period of time. If an employee retires and returns to work in the NHS within 1 month, his or her pension is normally suspended and any pension received must be repaid.

### Leaving the NHS Scheme

If an employee leaves the NHS Scheme he or she may transfer to private sector employers under the Transfer of Undertakings (Protection of Employment) Regulations as amended (TUPE). In such cases, although terms and conditions generally transfer under TUPE, pension benefits do not. The UK Government requires contractors in this situation to offer a 'broadly comparable pension, and its actuary department can issue a 'passport' confirming comparability. In practice, most NHS employees opt to freeze their NHS Pension Scheme membership and to take up the offer of a new pension with the private sector contractor.

## NHS terms of employment

Traditionally, pay and other terms and conditions of employment are determined centrally for all NHS employees. This is done through a system of Whitley councils and review bodies. Each occupational group within the NHS is covered by a different set of terms and conditions. For example, the terms for the administrative and clerical staff differ from those for medical and dental staff. These sets of employment terms have been supplemented over the years by collective negotiations, resulting in complex rules.

The advantage of a Whitley scheme is that the existence of nationwide terms facilitates mobility within the NHS. This is particularly so because previous service with other NHS employers is recognised in respect of certain terms of employment, for example, redundancy. However, set against this is the fact that the provisions contained in Whitley are so detailed as to be almost indecipherable to employees and employees alike.

## *Departure from Whitley*

Although NHS Trusts are entitled to adopt Whitley terms, they also have powers to employ staff on their own terms and conditions. As a result, many Trusts' contracts of employment have become a hybrid of Whitley and local terms. Whilst locally agreed terms and conditions tend to avoid the complexity of Whitley, there is one disadvantage: Trusts who have inherited staff on Whitley terms but who also have their own terms can find themselves employing staff on two different sets of terms and conditions.

## *Special health service terms of employment*

The Whitley Council had developed a number of special terms of employment which confer entitlements well in excess of those received by employees in the private sector. Key features of these are listed below.

### Sick pay

Staff are entitled to receive up to 6 months full pay and 6 months half pay in a period of 12 months, depending on the length of service.

### Continuity of service

Employment with any health service employer counts as 'reckonable service' even if there are breaks in service. However, for statutory purposes each NHS Trust and health authority is a separate employer except in the case of redundancy payments.

### Redundancy

Section 45 of the General Whitley Council Conditions confers very generous redundancy benefits on employees. A redundancy payment under the Whitley scheme is payable in much wider circumstances than under the statutory schemes. It is payable both for statutory redundancy and also for early retirement following organisational change.

Previous service with a health service authority is counted provided that there is no break exceeding 12 months. An employee loses the right to a redundancy payment if the employee unreasonably refuses an offer of suitable alternative employment with another health authority or NHS Trust.

### Early retirement
There are four classes of early retirement:

- ill health
- redundancy
- in the interests of the service
- for those over 50.

### Protection of earnings
Section 47 of the General Whitley Conditions provides for the protection of the earnings of any employee who is required to change posts following organisational change. Protection can be granted for a variety of time scales.

### Dismissal
Certain categories of staff such as doctors and dentists have the benefit of special dismissal procedures under Whitley.

## NHS Trusts
Under the 1990 Act, the first wave of 57 Trusts came into existence on 1 April 1991. These covered a range of services, including acute hospitals, community services, mental health, learning difficulties and ambulance services. By April 1994, after the fourth wave, the majority of units (some 400) had opted out of health authority management and had become NHS Trusts. The remainder became Trusts by 1996.

The main powers and responsibilities of Trust are as follows:

- to provide health services through contracts with health authorities and GP fundholders
- to manage NHS facilities vested in the Trust
- to generate income through commercial activities and private facilities
- to employ staff as necessary and determine their remunerations and terms of employment

- to determine its own management structure without needing approval from the health authorities, the NHS Executive or the DOH
- to provide high quality, accessible services to local communities
- to manage within financial allocations, and to benchmark costs and performance
- to recruit and retain staff who are suitably trained in providing complex and specialist services, and also to provide training and support to help staff deliver appropriate quality services
- to develop clinical governance arrangements to ensure quality
- to contribute to strategy and planning in the local HImPs (see entry).

### England
England has 8 Regions and 375 NHS Trusts, although the numbers are subject to change as mergers take place.

**N**

### Scotland
Scotland has 15 health boards and 35 NHS Trusts, a Common Services Agency, the Health Education Board for Scotland and the State Hospitals Board for Scotland, which are national organisations with responsibilities for associated services.

### Wales
Wales has 5 health authorities, 19 NHS Trusts and 2 health authorities specific to Wales (the Welsh Common Services Agency and the Health Promotion Authority for Wales).

### Northern Ireland
Northern Ireland has 4 area health boards and 19 health and social services Trusts.

### *Management of NHS Trusts*
Trust boards comprise a non-executive chairman and a chief executive together with up to five executive and non-executive directors.

The executive directors of a Trust hospital include:

- The Chief Executive
- The Director of Finance
- The Medical/Clinical Director
- The Head of Nursing
- One other director (e.g. of Human Resources, Corporate Affairs or Quality and Customer Services) or these roles combined with any of the above.

The chairperson and the non-executive directors are not full-time employees of the Trust. They are individuals with particular skills and management experience established outside of the Health Service. Two of the non-executive directors have to be local residents, and the remainder are appointed by the Secretary of State. In cases where the Trust has responsibilities for medical training, one of the non-executive directors has to be a person from the relevant medical school.

Trusts have a duty to comply with public health and patient health and safety regulations. Thus they are expected to comply with guidance on the notification of defects, of adverse reactions to drugs, and of communicable diseases. They also have to participate in emergency and contingency planning.

Unlike private hospitals, Trusts have to respond to quality standards demanded by the Department of Health (DOH) under such initiatives as the Patient's Charter. They have to provide statistical information required by the DOH for the purpose of monitoring. Trusts have to allow access to DOH and Home Office inspectors and to the Community Health Council.

### Trust management structure

The internal management of NHS Trusts may vary depending on the types of hospital and services provided. Trusts have full autonomy in deciding on their management structure. Most commonly, inpatient services in general hospital Trusts are grouped under specialties which are managed as directorates, e.g. medical directorate, child health directorate, etc. These may include one or several wards. Directorates are headed by a clinical director, who is assisted by a senior nurse and a business manager. The clinical director is a consultant within that specialty, with management responsibility to ensure that the

**N**

directorate performs in accordance with plans and objectives agreed by the chief executive and the Trust board. Directorates are given a budget to cover:

- staffing costs
- drugs and appliances
- funds to purchase other clinical support services, e.g. diagnostic and paramedical services
- hotel services including domestic, catering and portering and linen services
- building and maintenance
- administrative costs and supplies.

Other clinical services, e.g. radiography, pathology, physiological measurement and paramedical services, are grouped under functional lines and set up as business units in their own right, with their own budgets and income from the services they provide to the inpatient directorates and to those outside the Trust.

All non-clinical services are organised along functional lines (e.g. estate services, medical record administration, portering services), with functional heads accountable to a support services manager. Hotel services, such as domestic, linen and catering services (and more recently portering and security), have been subject to a programme of competitive tendering first introduced in 1983. All support services are expected to be managed along commercial lines in order to improve efficiency and cost-effectiveness. Trusts are expected to have more flexibility by introducing commercial and business systems prevalent in the business world.

### Community NHS Trusts

Community NHS Trusts provide such services as health visiting, school medical and nursing services, community chiropody, community dentistry, community nursing, child health, family planning, and well-women and well-men services. These generally have a directorate management structure, but directorates are formed along lines of geographical sectors, and directors may not necessarily be from the ranks of doctors. Community NHS Trusts also exist for mental illness and learning disability services. These have internal management arrangements which combine geographical sectorisation and specialty divisions.

# Nolan Report see Standards in public life

## Nurse, midwife and health visitor consultants

Plans for nurse, midwife and health visitor consultants were outlined in *Making a Difference: Strengthening the Nursing Midwifery and Health Visiting Contribution to Health and Healthcare* (DOH 1999b). The establishment of such posts is intended to help provide better outcomes for patients by improving services and quality, strengthening leadership and providing better career opportunities to help retain experienced, expert nurses, midwives and health visitors in practice. The first posts were filled in 2000, in various fields of practice.

Although job descriptions for consultant posts are tailored to local needs, each post has to be structured around four core functions:

- an expert practice function
- a professional leadership and consultancy function
- an education, training and development function
- a practice and service development, research and evaluation function.

Although it is recognised that the weight attached to each element will vary according to local circumstances, the posts are to be firmly practice based and at least 50% of the practitioner time must be spent in direct patient, client or community contact.

## Nurse practitioner

Although all nurses may refer to themselves as practitioners in the generic sense of those who practise their profession, the term 'nurse practitioner' usually has specific connotations. It is most frequently used by those who have undertaken specific preparation such as the RCN nurse practitioner programme. Such individuals will have usually extended their skills into areas such as differential diagnosis and direct referrals. However, because there is no legal or nationally accepted definition of the term and because considerable confusion and ambivalence over the nature and responsibilities of the role still exist, it is not safe to assume that use of the term necessarily implies anything other than a change in job title. The UKCC is addressing the issue as part of its work on higher level practice.

## Nurse prescribing

Nurse prescribing has been slowly rolling out in the NHS since the original proposals in the Cumberlege Report (Cumberlege 1986) on the review of community nursing, to the effect that 'the DHSS should agree to a limited list of items and simple agents which may be prescribed by nurses as part of a nursing care programme'.

In 1989, the Cumberlege Report was endorsed by the Crown Report (DOH 1989), the report of a working group chaired by Dr June Crown for the Department of Health. A recommendation was made that district nurses and health visitors should be eligible to prescribe from a limited nurses' formulary. In 1991, the UKCC issued guidelines relating to the educational needs of nurse prescribers and the national boards started to offer nurse prescribing courses. Nurse prescribing became law in the Prescription by Nurses, etc, Act 1992 and the first eight pilot sites were established for nurse prescribing – one for each health authority in England – in 1994. In 1998, central funding was announced for the national implementation of nurse prescribing although prescribing remains limited to those qualified and practising as district nurses and health visitors.

The Crown committee reconvened in 1999 to consider an extension to nurse prescribing and to extend nurse prescribing to other limited therapeutic areas by means of The Nurses Formulary (DOH 1999a). The National Plan contains proposals for an extension of nurse prescribing.

## Nursing

Probably the best and most widely known definition of nursing is that given by Virginia Henderson in 1996 in which she describes nursing thus:

> The unique function of the nurse is to assist the individual, sick or well, in the performance of those activities contributing to health or its recovery or to peaceful death that s/he would do unaided if s/he had the necessary strength, will or knowledge, and to do this in such a way as to

help her/him gain independence as rapidly as possible. (Henderson 1996)

It is important that any discipline has a clearly established paradigm, a world view and body of theory that directs its practice (Kuhn 1970). In nursing, this can be achieved by establishing the parameters of nursing practice, nursing being essentially an interpersonal, helping activity. In this context nursing involves one individual going out to another person or people with a helping intention, within a health and caring environment.

## Nursing and Midwifery Council

The Nursing and Midwifery Council is the body which replaced the UKCC (see entry) in April 2002 as the statutory regulatory body for nursing, midwifery and health visiting. It has 23 members – four nurses, four midwives and four health visitors each elected by the professions from the four countries for the UK (and 12 alternate members) and 11 lay numbers. The President is appointed by the Secretary of State for Health. Its functions are broadly similar to those of the four bodies it replaces – UKCC and National Boards for nursing, midwifery and health visiting (see entries).

**N**

### Office of the Information Commissioner

Subject to the provisions of the Freedom of Information Act, the Information Commissioner may conduct reviews of the decisions of public bodies in relation to requests for access to information. He may also carry out investigations at any time into the practices and procedures adopted by public bodies for the purposes of compliance with the Act. ✉ ① 📄 @

### Ombudsman see Health Service Commissioner

### Open and distance learning

Open and distance learning are terms which are often used interchangeably. Distance learning clearly describes learning that takes place away from a dedicated learning environment, such as a college, university or training department. It can refer to correspondence courses, computer based training and on-the-job learning. The term open learning, however, is used much more broadly and describes a philosophy which aims to open up opportunities for learning. So, although it is possible for open learning to be offered at a distance, not all distance learning is open.

Learning has never been more fashionable or accessible. There are very few professions that have not been touched by the government policies and practices which support lifelong learning. The assumption behind lifelong learning is that most of us learn most of the time – and are very good at it. We learn through our jobs, our hobbies, voluntary work, and our life and social situations. We learn through magazines, TV, radio and using the internet. We learn from our mistakes and through our achievements. All this is common sense. Learning is lifelong from the cradle to the grave.

However, not all experiences of learning are good. Many individuals had bad experiences at school, for example, and so people come to learning with preconceived ideas about what learning is or is not. Sometimes there is a need to unlearn what had already been learned. Many formal courses have previously concentrated on filling people up with knowledge, rather than developing thinking individuals who can think, act and learn for themselves. Open learning, therefore, is an approach to learning which recognises that:

- adults carry with them a wealth of knowledge and experience
- information, knowledge and ideas can nowadays be accessed easily and quickly
- some people need to break down their barriers to learning
- in all educational courses there should be an emphasis on the process of learning – that is, encouraging people to develop the skills they need to learn – rather than on the content – telling them what they should know
- people learn in different ways and most of us find it more rewarding to decide for ourselves how, what and where we will learn, than have other people decide for us.

The best open learning programmes start with where the learners are at the point of entry to the process, rather than where the tutor or institution thinks they should be. They aim to remove as many barriers to learning as possible: tutors do not see themselves as institutional gatekeepers. Open learning enables learners to choose the place, pace and timing of their study and places emphasis on the use of the professional's own experience of the learning process. Open learning, with its recognition that learning is lifelong, also promotes educational equality, by acknowledging that we all carry within us a wealth of experience and knowledge.

Open learning, with its emphasis on valuing learning wherever and however it happens, has the potential to bring a high degree of motivation, excitement and enthusiasm to the process. Individuals can bring all of their interests, values and passions to their professional development through this process. Open learning offers the chance to go out into the world and, through wide channels of information, learn and create new things.

Open learners are self-directed, autonomous professionals who think for themselves. They develop problem-solving approaches to their work and are able to evaluate their own performance and value their own theories and opinions. In short, open learning implies open people and an open society.

## Openness: the code of practice on openness in the NHS 1995

This code sets out the basic principles underlying public access to information about the NHS. It applies to Trusts, health authorities and individual registered practitioners such as doctors, dentists, pharmacists, nurses and midwives. Its governing principle is that the NHS should respond positively to requests for information. The code details the information which Trusts and HAs should make available in some form as a matter of good practice:

- information about what services are provided, the targets and standards set and results achieved, and the cost and effectiveness of the services
- details about important proposals on health policies or proposed changes in the way the services are delivered, including the reasons for those proposals
- details about important decisions on public health policies and decisions on changes in the delivery of services
- information about the way in which health services are managed and provided and who is responsible
- information about NHS communication with the public, such as details on public meetings, consultation procedures, suggestions and complaints systems
- information about how to contact Community Health Councils and the Health Service Commissioner (Ombudsman)
- information about how people can have access to their own personal records.

## A–Z guide

### Professions allied to medicine – professional colleges

There are profession-specific colleges for the professions allied to medicine (PAMs). Each undertakes, to varying degrees, education and training, examinations and standard setting functions. Contact details of the individual bodies can be found in Appendix 1.

### Partnerships with the voluntary sector

NHS organisations are permitted to share projects with the voluntary sector and in some cases to pool funding. There are a number of examples of this: for example, the Stroke Association (a voluntary body ⬚ ✉ ☎ ✍) has gained some research monies, and research is being carried out in a number of NHS centres across the UK. The Stroke Association has a number of staff trained to give specialist advice to individuals who have suffered strokes, and their families, and staff in the NHS can refer patients to this service. Other examples of partnerships are the range of local initiatives, based in the NHS, for which local people raise money in an organised way.

### ⬚ Patient Advocacy and Liaison Service

Following the proposals to abolish CHCs (see also CHCs) it is proposed that a Patient Advocacy and Liaison Service (PALS) be established in every Trust and PCT. The intention is that the new patient advocate team will be based inside the entrance of every hospital and serve as a welcoming and information point. Patient advocates will act as independent facilitators to handle patient concerns. In mental health and learning disability services, PALS will build on current specialist advocacy services, PALS will support complainants, with Citizens Advice Bureaux ensuring additional support. Current CHC funding will be redirected to fund PALS and other citizen empowerment mechanisms.

## Patients' Association

The Patients' Association is an independent charity pressing for the involvement of patients in decision making. The Association believes that patients should be involved as full partners in any decisions that affect them, be this with their GP or in policy decisions at government level. Its membership is made up of concerned individuals, health specific charities both large and small, health service organisations and private businesses. It runs a helpline that receives calls from people from all across the country who are often concerned at the care they or a relative have received, and the Association regularly receives correspondence from people giving their views of the quality of the health services. The Patients' Association remains independent as it does not rely on any single source of income and is non-political. The funding received comes from its membership, and from special events such as conferences. A National Lottery Grant has been of great support in developing the helpline.

## Patient's Charter

The Patient's Charter was published in 1991 and reviewed in 1995 and 1998. Charters are set at national level in England, Scotland, Wales and Northern Ireland and at health board or authority level. They make explicit the rights of individuals and the standards they can expect in healthcare. For example, everyone has the right to be registered with a GP or to receive healthcare on the basis of clinical need, regardless of the ability to pay. Standards, such as those relating to waiting time for ambulances or waiting time for initial assessment in accident and emergency units, are those which a patient can expect. The rights that all citizens can expect, together with national and local service guarantees and local targets, are also included.

In 2000, the Patient's Charter was replaced by *Your Guide to the NHS* (in England) (see entry), which sets out patients' rights and responsibilities.

## Patients' Forum

The Patients' Forum is a network of over 60 national and regional organisations with a concern for the healthcare interests of patients and their carers. It aims to provide a forum for its members to promote patient and carer representation in the health policy process and to exchange information and ideas. ✉ ☏ ☞

## ⧉ Patient forum

A patient forum will be established in every Trust and PCT with half the members being drawn from local patient groups and voluntary organisations and the remainder drawn randomly from respondents to the Trust's annual survey. The forum will be supported by the new PALS and will have the right to visit and inspect any aspects of the Trust's care at any time. The forum will also elect a representative to the Trust Board.

## ⧉ Patient Information Forum

The Patient Information Forum (PIF) was created at the beginning of 1997 to act as a support and information network for people responsible for producing patient information in the NHS. PIF promotes and supports the role of patient information managers/officers mainly, but not exclusively, in NHS Trust settings. It produces a newsletter and a directory of people working in the information field and holds conferences and workshops. PIF is preparing guidelines on writing patient information. ✉

## Personal Medical Services pilots

The NHS (Primary Care) Act 1997 allows an NHS Trust, an NHS employee, a qualifying body and suitably experienced medical practitioners capable of providing primary health care to submit proposals to provide services under a pilot and contract with the health authority to do so. These are known as Personal Medical Services (PMS). They are voluntary schemes offered as an alternative to the traditional GP model. They are intended to provide services which are more sensitive to local needs and can manage present shortcomings, for example, the shortage of GPs. Models vary, for example, GPs and nurses working together, nurse led schemes and salaried GPs working for community trusts. Some target specific groups such as the homeless and the elderly. 85 had been established by 1999 in Scotland and England and rapid roll out is expected.

## Portfolios see Profiles and portfolios

## Portfolio careers

Changing contexts need flexible professionals. Security of employment in the health service is a thing of the past and no professional is immune. Movement through recognised hierarchies has been replaced by pathways of progression across, downwards, diagonally or upwards. Professionals need to adopt a portfolio approach to both career choices and developmental activities. A portfolio approach to career development and progression requires a different mind set – one which values every piece of experience as a contribution to future roles. Portfolio career development encourages a 'pick and mix' approach towards skills and knowledge, rather than being driven by the job title. This diversity can open up a range of new prospects. Warmly espoused by Charles Handy (Handy 1995), portfolio people are those who do not intend to stay in one career all their lives – even if that were an option – but plan to use their marketable skills, product or service in a variety of settings. Portfolio careers are more circular than traditional patterns of employment and have a different set of rewards, which may include some in kind, some in money, some in freedom to organise one's own time and a consequential satisfaction in experiencing a range of different opportunities.

## Preceptorship

**P**

Preceptorship is part of the continuum of clinical supervision. Although the term is open to different interpretations and is often used interchangeably with mentorship, within the healthcare professions it is used most frequently in relation to the period of support for the newly qualified nurse, midwife or health visitor recommended as good practice by the UKCC.

The UKCC recommend that: 'as good practice, all newly registered nurses, midwives and health visitors should be provided with a period of support, where possible under the guidance of a preceptor, for approximately the first 4 months of professional practice' (UKCC 1995). It is further recommended that preceptors receive specific preparation and that the exact model of support be worked out to suit the needs of the preceptor and preceptee concerned. Many places now have preceptorship programmes in place for the newly qualified, although provision across the UK remains uneven.

## PREP

PREP is the acronym given to the continuing professional development standards and requirements for nurses, midwives and health visitors, established by the UKCC. PREP stands for Post Registration Education and Practice. There are a number of elements to the requirements, some of which are statutory and some of which are advisory. The statutory elements, which came into force in 1995, are enshrined in the 'PREP rules' (HMSO 1995). They are that in every 3-yearly registration period, practitioners wishing to maintain their registration must:

- complete a minimum of 5 days or 35 hours of learning activity relevant to their work
- maintain a personal professional profile of their learning activity
- comply with any request from the UKCC to audit how the requirements have been met
- have worked in some capacity by virtue of their nursing, midwifery or health visiting qualification during the previous 5 years for a minimum of 750 hours, or undertaken an approved return to practice programme.

An individual's UKCC registration will lapse if he or she fails to meet the above requirements, which means that the individual will be unable to work as a registered nurse, midwife or health visitor.

## Primary care groups

Primary care groups (PCGs) bring together family doctors, community nurses and others and were established to commission NHS services to meet systematically defined health needs within communities of 100 000–200 000 people. They contribute to the local HImPs and have a budget reflecting their population's share of the available resources for hospital and community health services, the general medical services cash-limited budget and resources for prescribing. The groups have the opportunity to become free standing Primary Care Trusts (PCTs) (see entry). They have a responsibility to reduce inequalities through integrating health and social care and involving consumers, whilst moving towards evidence based practice.

Their responsibilities are to:

- contribute to the Health Authority's Health Improvement Programme
- promote the health service for their population
- monitor performance against service agreement with Trusts
- develop primary care, and
- integrate primary and community services more fully and work more closely with social services on both the planning and delivery of services.

There are four levels of PCG responsibility, as follows:

- *Level 1*: to support the health authority in commissioning care for its population, acting in an advisory capacity
- *Level 2*: to take devolved responsibility for managing the budget for healthcare in their area, as part of the health authority
- *Level 3*: to become established as freestanding bodies, accountable to the health authority for commissioning care
- *Level 4*: as level 3 but with the additional responsibility for the provision of community health services for the population.

The boards have 11–13 members, made up of 4–7 GPs, 1–2 community nurses, the PCG Chief Executive, a health authority non-executive member, a social services nominee and 2 lay members.

## Primary Care Trusts

Primary Care Trusts (PCTs) are free standing statutory bodies established as a result of the Health Act 1999. They started running from 1 April 2000. They will undertake many of the functions currently undertaken by health authorities, such as commissioning services, investing in primary and community care and improving the health of the local population. Their aim will be to improve the health of the community through the development of primary and community health services and the commissioning of secondary care services. To do this they will work collaboratively with patients, users, carers, GPs and other local organisations. There will be two levels of PCT – level 1

Trusts will undertake the range of services described above and level 2 PCTs will, in addition, be able to provide services themselves, such as running community hospitals. They will have their own budgets and be held to account by the local health authority for their performance in commissioning and providing healthcare.

## Primary Immunodeficiency Association

The Primary Immunodeficiency Association (PiA) provides support to patients and families affected by a primary immunodeficiency. It aims to advance education about these conditions within the medical profession, among patients and their families, and in the general public, thus promoting improvements in diagnosis and provision of medical care. ✉ ☎ 📄 @ 🔗

## Primary legislation

Primary legislation refers to the legislation enshrined in Acts of Parliament (see Legislative process of a government bill).

## Private Finance Initiative

The Private Finance Initiative (PFI) is a major change in the methods of procurement in the public sector. It also requires a significant shift in perception by both the public sector and the private sector. It can be applied to the provision of new accomodation or refurbishment of existing buildings, or to the provision of medical equipment and information management and technology (IM&T) systems.

Under traditional methods of procurement, when a hospital is to be built using public capital, the NHS Trust would draw up a detailed specification. The private sector body would build the hospital to that specification. The Trust would pay for the hospital that was being built, with final payments following its completion. It would have required an asset – the building – which would be on the Trust's balance sheet. Once the building was completed and any defects dealt with, the private company would have no other involvement. The NHS body would be responsible for the subsequent maintenance, repair and operation of the building and the provision of the necessary support services. It may choose to contract these out but that would be a separate exercise from the acquisition of the building.

Under PFI, the NHS body is not acquiring an asset but instead is purchasing a service. The provider of that service is likely to be a consortium of companies led by a company specially formed for that purpose, usually described as a Special Purpose Vehicle (SPV). The NHS body contracts with the SPV typically under what is called a design, build, finance and operate (DBFO) contract. The consortium will consist of the building company and the service providers. The clinical services will be provided by the NHS body.

The SPV will be responsible for the whole life costs of the building and the provision of agreed support services during the period of its contract with the NHS body. That provides incentives to the consortium to design the building in the most efficient way, to reduce the need for maintenance, and to ensure efficiency in the provision of the support services. Until the hospital is built and is available for use by the NHS body, no payment is made. Then unitary power will become payable, usually on a monthly or quarterly basis, representing payment for the services. The price will be predetermined, subject only to indexation (usually in accordance with the retail price index (RPI)) and to variation in accordance with a detailed change mechanism in the contract. Payment will be subject to measures such as availability of bed spaces and performance measures in relation to the support services. There may also be some measures linked to volume and usage.

A PFI scheme must deliver value for money. It must be affordable and it must be bankable. One of its characteristics will be the significant transfer of risk to the private sector during the construction phase and during the operational phase, which will be reflected in the payment mechanism. Risk should be transferred to the person best able to manage it, which is why transfer of volume risk to the private sector has not, so far, been a major feature in hospital schemes.

## Professional conduct and discipline

Many of those working in the healthcare professions are required, before they may practise, to be registered with a professional or regulatory body. Currently, for example, doctors must register with the General Medical Council (GMC), nurses, midwives and health visitors with the United Kingdom Central

Council for Nursing, Midwifery and Health Visiting (UKCC), and those professions supplementary to medicine with the Council for Professions Supplementary to Medicine (CPSM).

Whilst separate statutes currently govern the regulation of each of the three groups referred to above, it is the Government's intention, in accordance with the Health Act 1999, to bring about an effective fusion of the individual systems of regulation which have applied to date. Once the Health Act is in place it will be open to the Secretary of State, by secondary legislation, to determine the regulatory issues for all professions 'concerned (wholly or partly) with the physical or mental health of individuals'. Distinction is drawn between the professions of medicine, dentistry, pharmacy, optics, osteopathy, chiropracty and nursing, midwifery and health visiting, and the other professions. Regulation of the former group of professions may merely be modified by the Secretary of State, whereas regulation of the other professions (which may include some not previously the subject of regulation, for example, carers) may be undertaken by the Secretary of State from scratch.

Regulation of professions includes the setting of standards of conduct for those practising. Written codes of conduct are commonly issued to members as an advance warning of conduct that would not be viewed as acceptable. It is important for health professionals to realise that their conduct, both within their professional practice and outside it, is regulated. Hence a person found guilty of shop-lifting or excessive discipline of his or her own child, for example, may face an allegation of unprofessional conduct and by virtue of this, a threat to his or her right to practise.

The underlying purpose of a regulatory code of professional conduct is to protect the members of the public with whom professionals come into contact. It also reassures those members of the public that the overall standard of conduct, in life, of the members of the profession reaches a uniformly acceptable level.

It is likely that, with the enactment of the Health Act, greater uniformity of regulation of healthcare professions will take place, and it is greatly to be welcomed that the Act is likely to lead to regulation, for the first time, of the many careers dealing with those who are perhaps the most vulnerable members of society.

## Professional development see Portfolio careers

## Professional self-regulation

For most professions, self (as opposed to externally imposed) regulation was a hard won battle and passionately argued as serving the public good. 'Self' can refer to the individual or the profession as a whole. Maintaining an active self-regulatory process is part of the duty of every practitioner and must be properly understood and regularly re-negotiated in order to maintain the special relationship that has been developed over time with the public.

Regulation is the means by which order, consistency and control are brought to a profession. The goal of an effective regulatory system should be to protect the public. Regulation in its widest sense refers to all the standards set in relation to a profession – not merely those relating to professional conduct or discipline. It should encompass the standards for education leading to registration, standards for registration itself, standards for maintaining registration and standards for the removal or limitation of registration. The register, therefore, is at the heart of the process as an instrument of public protection.

As society changes, so does the relationship between the individuals within it and the systems for governing it. Many of the recent changes in the health service directly impact on the healthcare professions and their systems of self-regulation. The current Government is committed to strengthening the existing systems of regulation by ensuring that they are open, responsive and accountable (DOH 1997).

Self-regulation is an accountability based system, carrying with it specific responsibilities. Such responsibilities are frequently set out in codes of conduct or behaviour, for example, the code of conduct produced by the UKCC which applies to all registered nurses, midwives and health visitors.

Self-regulation activities include self- and peer-review, clinical supervision, systematic practice development, credentialling, practice privileges, professional audit and portfolio development.

## Profiles and portfolios

The terms profile and portfolio have become part of the healthcare language, particularly but not exclusively for nurses, midwives and health visitors. The idea originally came from the American higher education system. The idea stems from two educational theories about the way that adults learn – that is *experiential learning* and *reflective practice*. Experiential learning, or learning from experience, can happen when you are directly involved in a situation, but it does not happen by accident. Learning takes place from participation in the situation, as well as from taking time to reflect on what took place. The notion that people could learn from experience and reflection meant that there needed to be a way of recording this activity. The result was a profile or portfolio.

The terms profile and portfolio are often used interchangeably. Strictly speaking, the term portfolio should be used when referring to a wider ranging collection of evidence about learning, which might include personal and professional interests. A profile is much more specific – a selection of evidence for a specific purpose to present to a specific audience. An example of this is the personal professional profile which nurses, midwives and health visitors are required by the UKCC to keep, in order to meet their re-registration requirements (see PREP). To some extent the term used is irrelevant. It is, however, important when an individual is required to keep a profile or portfolio that its purpose is clear and that the expectations about content and style, for example, are unambiguous. Profiles and portfolios are now a common learning tool in all fields of education and practice. Generally speaking, whichever term is used, there are common characteristics. Profiles and portfolios:

- value experience as a source of learning
- provide a storehouse of evidence of experience, learning and achievements
- encourage personal and professional development.

There are a number of key points to remember when completing and maintaining a profile or portfolio:

- Although an individual will have to write in the profile, it is not usually the writing style or ability that is being judged. What has been learned is far more important.
- It must contain evidence of learning. Evidence is more than just a record of having attended a study day, for example.

It needs to include the aims and objectives of the day, what you learned from attending, how it was applied to your professional practice and an evaluation of how successful, or otherwise, that was.

- There is no point in collecting details of your learning activities unless these can be supported by direct or indirect evidence.
- A profile can be organised in any way that makes sense to the individual concerned, providing the information contained can be easily retrieved. Check that the format meets the expectations of whoever may be asking for the contents.
- Start to build the profile from the place which makes most sense to you – do not try and complete it all at once. Start with the section which seems easiest or most relevant.
- A profile is a personal document and it should be established at the outset whether any of the sections will be needed for perusal by others and why.
- The contents will need to be reviewed from time to time and unnecessary material weeded out.
- Reviewing content can be a useful way of demonstrating how much has been achieved over time (Hull & Redfern 1996).

## Project 2000

**P**

Project 2000 is the name given to the reforms in nursing and midwifery education which took place in the 1980s. The changes were designed to prepare practitioners more effectively for the professional practice of nursing, midwifery and health visiting in relation to projected health needs in the 1990s and beyond. A number of key changes emerged: the move towards one level of nurse; programmes of preparation divided into an 18-month common foundation programme and an 18-month branch programme, with subsequent registration in either adult, children's, mental health or learning disabilities nursing; the need for a comprehensive framework for post registration education (which subsequently became the PREP project); and supernumerary status for students. The latter recommendation, together with the move into higher education, away from hospital based schools of nursing, subsequently attracted criticism from some quarters.

In 1999, a UKCC Commission for Nursing and Midwifery Education, chaired by Sir Len Peach (UKCC 1999), found that, although in the main, the Project 2000 changes were working satisfactorily, substantial modifications were needed in some areas to ensure greater emphasis on the competencies to be expected of registered practitioners. Steps are being taken through pilot schemes to address these shortfalls.

## Protocols

Protocols refer to written plans which specify the procedures to be followed in, for example, giving a practical examination, conducting research, or providing care for a particular condition. Also referred to as *clinical guidelines*, they are increasingly used for ensuring quality, continuity and consistency in the delivery of care. They provide a checklist for clinicians to ensure that they are providing the best and most appropriate treatment for each individual patient. They often set out a treatment/care pathway and offer different options which can be taken according to the patient's progress and preferences. The guidelines are based on the best available evidence, which may be deduced from research, best practice or traditional treatment. Whilst the preparation of guidelines has rested with particular professional or multiprofessional interest groups, NICE and the Clinical Standards Board for Scotland will increasingly assume a coordinating role for the work.

## Public Interest Disclosure Act 1999

This is known as the 'Whistleblower's Act' – an Act which came into force in July 1999 giving greater legal protection to employees who blow the whistle on wrongdoing or malpractice in the workplace. For the first time this legislation gives some support to those who have the courage to expose wrong doing, providing the individual reasonably believes the allegations to be true, does not make the disclosure for personal gain, or does not contravene the Official Secrets Act. The new law is an extension of the Government's moves against the 'gagging' clauses which are in some individuals' contracts. A worker may take his or her employer to tribunal for any detriment (dismissal, redundancy, etc.) after the worker blows the whistle on matters relating to:

- a criminal offence
- a breach of legal obligation (e.g. duty of care)
- where the health and safety of the employee is likely to be endangered
- a miscarriage of justice
- environmental damage.

...................................................................................................................

P

# A–Z guide

## Qualifications and Curriculum Authority

The Qualifications and Curriculum Authority (QCA) is a public body responsible for promoting quality and coherence in education and training. Its remit ranges from early years to higher level vocational qualifications. It is responsible for ensuring that the curriculum and qualifications available to young people and adults are of high quality, coherent and flexible. It helps to raise national standards of achievement through promoting greater access to education and training, improving opportunities for lifelong learning, creating ways of giving credible national recognition for all learners and encouraging greater achievements. ✉ ☾ 🖺

## Quality

Over the last decade, issues surrounding quality within the NHS have risen to prominence due to an increased concentration on guaranteeing value for money and moving the focus for service provision to improving the experience of patients and clients. Quality has been put at the heart of the NHS business in that it forms the central theme of clinical governance.

Quality in the past attracted a somewhat mundane image. Many discussions on the subject would quote at length from Donabedian and work to the mantra of structure, process and outcome. While this can be a very useful framework for assessing and determining the quality of services, it can be argued that the establishment of clinical governance brings new meaning to the development of quality.

Quality will now be assessed, measured and monitored through a variety of local, regional and national means. NHS Trusts, for example, will be responsible for ensuring that the quality of services they offer improves year on year. This will be achieved through the improved collection of data on a series of clinical indicators and the establishment of service standards and protocols covering medicine, nursing and the other clinical professions. A new statutory duty of quality will be enshrined in law, where the chief executive and his responsible officers will have to sign statements assuring patients and clients that the quality of services is of a particular standard and systems are in place to ensure this. Accountability lies specifically with the chief executive.

Increasingly, systems are being put into place regionally and nationally to monitor the effectiveness of Trust quality systems. This national framework includes the National Institute of Clinical Effectiveness (England and Wales) and the Clinical Standards Board (Scotland) which will be responsible for national standard setting through national service frameworks and clinical guidelines. Expected standards of care will then be disseminated to Trusts who will ensure that these are implemented, forming the basis of an increased emphasis on evidence based care. The effectiveness of this standard setting will be monitored by the Commission for Health Improvement (CHI). In the majority of cases the role of the CHI will be to determine that Trusts are working to a required standard. In some instances the CHI will be required to go into a Trust and implement systems to rectify shortfalls in quality as these are identified.

While some clinicians have portrayed these arrangements as 'being watched by big brother', there is little doubt that the renewed emphasis on quality has been welcomed by the majority of clinical professionals. Quality can now be seen as a positive feature of health services which can progressively be developed with the official sanction of government. The question of resources always arises, although many organisations are finding that they can reassign existing resources to go some way towards enabling them to measure and monitor quality effectively.

Finally, clear signals have been sent to the NHS suggesting that utilising a systematised approach to quality or gaining external accreditation is increasingly favoured. To this end, independent systems are increasingly providing health service organisations with a framework to assure outside agencies that they are providing high quality care, while working to develop the quality of their services over time.

# Queen's Nursing Institute

The Queen's Nursing Institute (QNI) exists to improve the quality of nursing healthcare to the community so that people can receive the best attention and advice available to deal with the health needs of modern life. Amongst other things, the organisation provides financial support and professional development for community nurses and supports a wide range of nurse led practice initiatives, including substance abuse, health in schools and sexual health. ✉ ① 🖱

Q

## Record keeping

Accurate and effective record keeping by all healthcare professionals is a vital part of responsible professional practice. The following summary, based on UKCC guidance, has relevance for all healthcare professionals:

- Record keeping is an integral part of professional practice.
- Good record keeping is a mark of safe and skilled practitioners.
- Records should not include abbreviations, jargon, meaningless phrases, irrelevant speculation and offensive statements.
- Records should be written in terms that the patient or client can easily understand.
- By auditing records, the standard of the record can be assessed and used to identify areas of improvement and staff development.
- Any entry made in a record must be identified clearly.
- Patients and clients have a right of access to records held about them.
- Each practitioner's contribution to records should be seen as of equal importance.
- Each practitioner has a duty to protect the confidentiality of the patient or client record.
- The principle of confidentiality must be equally honoured in computer held records.
- Patients and clients should own their own healthcare records as far as is appropriate and as long as they are happy to do so.
- The use of records in research should be approved by the local research ethics committee.
- Professional judgement must be used in deciding what is relevant and what should be recorded.

- Records should be written clearly and in such a manner that the text cannot be erased.
- Records should be factual, consistent and accurate.
- Records should be made on the assumption that they may be scrutinised at some point.
- Good record keeping helps to protect the welfare of patients and clients.

(Based on *Guidelines for Records and Record Keeping* UKCC 1998b.)

## Reflective practice

Reflective practice has become increasingly important for the practice based professions as the value of critical reflection or critical incident analysis has been recognised. Its chief proponent is Donald Schon who argued that the application of text book principles and solutions to a given problem does not work for the complex problems which have to be dealt with by competent professionals (Schon 1987). Instead, innovative and creative actions need to be designed for each unique problem. In this way links are established between thinking and doing. Schon believes that different professions share common characteristics, as follows:

- Professionals face complex problems in their day-to-day work. There are no definitively right or wrong answers but only good and not so good ones.
- When making decisions, professionals draw on a knowledge base which is broad, deep and multifaceted.
- The context in which professionals use their knowledge and skills is very important.
- Professional knowledge is not just about having expert skills.
- It is often difficult for professionals to say or write about what they know and how they use their knowledge.

R

Schon talks about 'reflection-on-action' – thinking about what you or colleagues did in a particular situation and why specific decisions/actions were taken – and also about 'reflection-in-action' – undertaken during practice when applying knowledge from past events to the situation in hand. The process of systematic reflection is a valuable learning tool and will help individuals both learn about themselves and advance their personal and professional knowledge and skills.

## ▨ Registered Nursing Home Association

The Registered Nuring Home Association (RNHA) was formed in 1968. Essentially, it is an association run for its members, who are nursing home owners. Its elected national committee, led by a chairman and vice chairman, determines overall policy, with individual committee members taking on responsibility for over-seeing and driving forward particular activities.

Members have a major opportunity to influence policy through their local branches and by attending and voting at the national conference.

A small head office team of permanent staff, based in Birmingham and led by a nursing home owner, implements RNHA policy and ensures continuity of service to members. Above all, the aim is to ensure a balance between representing members' interests at a national level and supporting their work in delivering high quality nursing care at a local level. ⊠ ① 🗎 ⌐

## Registered nursing homes see Teaching nursing homes

## ▨ Research into Ageing

Research into Ageing is a biomedical research organisation that funds biomedical research into ageing. ⊠ ① 🗎 @ ⌐

## Revenue

Revenue is the term given to money which is used for things which are regular items in an organisation's budget, such as staff wages, utility (gas, electric, etc.) bills and maintenance contracts. When spending capital money, it is important to take into account any revenue money that will be required to support that capital spend, for example, when spending capital on a big piece of equipment, one should carefully weigh up the cost of paying the staff to use it. (See also Capital.)

## Risk management
### Definition
Risk management and decision making are the assessing and balancing of negative and positive outcomes and are at the heart of quality care. The Oxford Modern English Dictionary defines

risk as: 'Chance or possibility of danger, loss, injury or other adverse outcome'. What is defined as risk is largely determined by social and cultural responses (Douglas 1992). An individual's own value base will influence his or her attitude to risk and the perspective of a keen diver or mountaineer will therefore differ from that of someone who is less adventurous.

## Organisational culture

Whilst individual professionals are accountable practitioners, decision making is not conducted in a vacuum. The culture of the organisation is influential: one that operates a culture of blame rather than support is likely to encourage defensive practice aimed at protecting staff rather than promoting patient autonomy.

## Policies and procedures

Risk taking should be supported by clear guidance and policy. Policies should reflect the organisation's risk-taking philosophy, for example, the promotion of patient autonomy. Risk policies should be clearly written, evidence based and demonstrate appreciation of the likely risks. Care provision may otherwise fail. For example, an observation policy that has no mechanism for continuing observation whilst a mental health patient is off the ward, fails to appreciate the risks inherent in providing departmentalised care and provides opportunity for absconding and possible self-harm.

## Practice

Risk assessment and management of risk is an ongoing process and requires an evaluative, reflective approach such as that used in care mapping. Use of care pathways and risk mapping is an acknowledged 'powerful weapon both minimising clinical risk and neutralising the increasing threat of litigation' (Smith 1999). Professional practice involves competing demands of professional accountability and client autonomy in addition to the responsibilities as an employee to comply with guidance and policy. Such dilemmas may lead to the avoidance of risk taking, which in turn may underline a client or patient's autonomy and ability to achieve potential. Risk avoidance is as much a decision as risk taking. Weighing up and balancing conflicting interests and justifying the decision made is an integral part of professional practice. It is not about creating a risk free environment, but about being able to justify your risk decisions, based on personal professional competence, an evaluative, reflective approach and good record keeping.

### Record keeping

Integral to good practice is good record keeping, not least because it is essential to risk management. Good quality record keeping underpins the delivery of care by promoting prompt communication and evaluation. Whilst guidance (DOH 1999b) requires the implementation of record-keeping systems, there is currently no national standard on the content of a record. The quality of record keeping will affect the quality for practice as well as proving the evidence to justify decisions.

### Risk and the law

There is no legal concept of risk. The law does, however, provide frameworks for analysing decisions. A decision may be challenged on the grounds that it was negligent. To establish a claim for damages for negligence a person must show what duty of care was owed to him or her, that it has been breached and that, in consequence, harm that was reasonably foreseeable and that can be compensated has occurred. If harm has occurred but was not caused by the breach, then there can be no claim of compensation.

### Standard of care

The standard of care is judged against whether a responsible body of professional opinion would have made the same decision (Bolam v Frien Hospital Management Committee 1957 1 WLR 582) and further that the decision is capable of logical analysis (Bolitho v City and Hackney Health Authority 1997 2 ALL ER 771). Even if there is no claim for damages, an individual's professional practice may come under scrutiny in other ways such as disciplinary hearings, complaint, inquest or public enquiry.

Although the courts do consider an organisation's mechanism for managing risk, claims or damages are most likely to be decided by the actions of individual practitioners. This is because the standard of care focuses primarily on individual professional practice rather than on organisational structure and systems. However, as clinical governance, record management systems and audit have increasing impact, managers and chief executives may also come under scrutiny for poor decision-making management systems.

## Royal College of Midwives

The Royal College of Midwives (RCM) is the trades union and professional organisation for midwives, with over 37 000 members. It provides a range of trade union expertise in areas such as professional representation, advice on employment matters, representation at industrial tribunals and health and safety monitoring in the workplace. It also provides professional support, advice and information, publications, professional development and guidance and leadership for its members. Working through its branches, RCM boards and council, the College offers a strong and coherent voice on midwifery and related issues at national and international level. ✉ ☏ 📄

## Royal College of Nursing

The Royal College of Nursing (RCN) is the world's largest union of nurses, with over 300 000 members. It is the second largest trades union in the UK outside the Trades Union Congress and is the fastest growing. The RCN is a major contributor to the development of nursing practice and standards of care, is a provider of higher education and is a registered charity. It promotes the interests of nurses and patients on a wide range of issues by working with governments, MPs, other unions, professional and statutory bodies and voluntary organisations. It is the voice of UK nursing abroad and is represented on many European, Commonwealth and international bodies, including the International Council of Nurses.

The RCN offers a wide range of services to its members including advice on pay and conditions, legal and labour relations representation, professional advice and counselling, courses, seminars and conferences, and up-to-date information on developments in nursing and healthcare. The RCN Council is the RCN's governing body, made up of 24 democratically elected members representing 14 English regions, Northern Ireland, Scotland and Wales and the College's student membership.

## Royal College of Speech and Language Therapists

The Royal College of Speech and Language Therapists (RCSLT) is the professional body for speech and language therapists in the UK. It is responsible for the promotion and maintenance of high standards in the education, clinical practice and ethical conduct of speech and language therapists.

## Royal Institute of Public Health and Hygiene and Society of Public Health

The Royal Institute of Public Health and Hygiene and Society of Public Health (RIPHH & SPH) is a not-for-profit, non-governmental organisation, registered as a charity in the UK. The aim of the Royal Institute is to promote the advancement of public health and hygiene for people of all ages at home, school, work or recreation. It seeks to advance and develop public health, preventative medicine and hygiene, especially personal, domestic or industrial hygiene, and public education about these matters.

## Royal Pharmaceutical Society of Great Britain

The Royal Pharmaceutical Society of Great Britain (RPSGB) is the professional organisation for pharmacy. It works in a number of different ways to promote development of higher standards of practice and to safeguard public health. Its key roles are:

- keeping the professional register (approximately 43 000 pharmacists)
- supervising education and training
- working nationwide with a programme of professional, educational and social activity
- raising standards
- guarding public safety
- publishing worldwide.

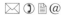

## Royal Society of Health

The Royal Society of Health (RSH) is a charity founded in 1876. The society aims to:

- improve the quality and dignity of human life worldwide
- promote continuous improvement of health and safety through education, communication and scientific research.

It is an awarding body offering examinations in areas such as meat inspection, food hygiene, oral hygiene, nutrition, pest control, environmental protection, counselling and health and safety. It also offers a variety of UK conferences on health related matters.

The RSH is governed by an elected council of 28 members drawn from a wide range of healthcare professionals, environmental health workers, social workers, nutritionists and others working in medicine and health. ✉ ① 📄 🖱

## Royal Society of Medicine

The Royal Society of Medicine (RSM) is an independent, apolitical organisation. Its aims are:

- to provide a broad range of educational activities for doctors, dentists and veterinary surgeons, including students of those disciplines, and for allied healthcare professionals
- to promote an exchange of information and ideas on the science, practice and organisation of medicine both within the health professions and through responsible, informed public opinion.

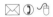

R

## Sainsbury Centre for Mental Health

The Sainsbury Centre for Mental Health was established in 1985 to develop effective ways of delivering mental health services. It seeks to influence national policy formulation through its research and development findings. It has a strong national reputation for innovation and excellence in its work, which incorporates research and evaluation, development and training, and communications and publications. Its staff include those with mental health backgrounds – as service users and practitioners. ✉ 🖰

## SCOTCATS see Credit Accumulation and Transfer Schemes

## Scottish Association of Health Councils see Community Health Councils

## Scottish Health Information Network

The aim of the Scottish Health Information Network (SHINE) is to ensure the best possible access to the knowledge base of healthcare through supporting activities and developments in library and information services in Scotland. Its objectives include:

- to seek opportunities to inform and influence relevant policy-making and funding bodies on issues relating to healthcare library and information services
- to act as a forum for exchange of views and information
- to promote collaborative effort and partnership between the healthcare library and information services in all sectors This will include sharing of resources and expertise, shared problem solving, and networking by both electronic and other means

- to facilitate quality improvement in healthcare library and information services through promotion of recognised/approved guidelines and standards.

Membership consists of four categories: personal, institutional, associate and life. ✏

## Scottish Parliament

The Scotland Act 1998 legalised Scottish devolution. Work previously undertaken by the Scottish Office and other Scottish Departments passed to the Scottish Parliament, under the guidance of a First Minister and a team of ministers who manage the Scottish Executive. The Scottish Parliament is responsible for the day-to-day running of the NHS, public health and mental health issues, the education and training (but not regulation) of health professionals and the service conditions of GPs and NHS staff. The Parliament also has powers to legislate on a wide ranging set of issues, including health.

## Scottish Qualifications Authority

The Scottish Qualifications Authority (SQA) was set up in April 1997 following the merger of the Scottish Vocational and Education Council (SCOTVEC) and the Scottish Examining Board (SEB). Unlike QCA, it has both accrediting and awarding body responsibilities.

## Seamless care/interagency working

The NHS White Paper *The New NHS: Modern, Dependable* (DOH 1997) gave birth to a large number of initiatives with a view to bringing the Health Service into the new millennium as a 'modern and dependable' service. Some of these initiatives are not new but extensions of policy that go back at least to the NHS Act 1977. One of these areas relates to the interface between health and social services. Section 22 of the 1977 Act states: 'In exercising their respective functions, Health Authorities...and Local Authorities shall co-operate with one another to secure and advance the health and welfare of the people of England and Wales'.

Clause 19 of the Health Act 1999 contains an explicit duty on Health Authorities, special Health Authorities, Primary Care Trusts and NHS Trusts to cooperate with each other, and

S

Section 22 of the NHS Act 1977 is to be extended by the Health Bill to impose a duty of cooperation on PCTs and NHS Trusts with local authorities. Further to this, successive policy guidances have stressed the need for local authorities and health service bodies to collaborate and coordinate their activities.

So why is this important? The simple answer is that policy dictates that care for every individual shall pass seamlessly to different agencies at different stages of care, depending upon the care provided by relevant agencies. All the resources available should be effectively and efficiently employed in the best interests of the patient.

Primarily, the Health Service is responsible for 'healthcare'. It is easy to see how 'healthcare' applies to someone who is taken into hospital because they are acutely ill. However, past a certain point in that care the patient will be well enough to be discharged from hospital from which point, however, they may need further care. This could be 'social care', which is provided by local authority social services, or a mixture of 'healthcare' and 'social care', depending, for example, upon the age, condition and dependency levels of the patient concerned.

The difference between health and social care is important because healthcare is defined as being 'free at the point of delivery', whereas social care need not be. In some cases, local authorities are obliged to charge for services that they provide, subject to exemptions for clients on low incomes or resources. It is important for the client and his or her family, both from a care and a resources viewpoint, to know what is going to happen to them, when this will happen, who will be caring for them and the financial consequences.

To work properly, in the best interests of that patient, all this requires a high degree of collaboration and discussion between the responsible agencies. Patients – especially old and frail patients – need to know and have comfort that there will be a seamless transition between the care provided in the hospital and wherever they go on to next, whether that be to their own home, with or without support, or to a nursing home or residential home. It should always be the case that no-one in need of continuing or further care (within the NHS guidance HSC (95)8) leaves or is discharged from hospital without a proper package of care which has been agreed between a multidisciplinary team following a full assessment of the patient's needs. Whether the necessary cooperation to produce such care packages always takes place or is always available is open to question.

The duty to cooperate referred to above may improve effective collaboration between health and social services and other relevant agencies, for example, the voluntary sector, but with some relationships this may only follow effective enforcement of the duty.

Under the Health Act there are new powers, set out in regulations, to pool budgets and maximise new resources, but these will only prove useful tools to those health and local authorities who have a history of joint working and service alignment. As for the others, good practice may only be implemented and a seamless service become a reality following mandatory guidance and enforcement.

## Secondary legislation

Secondary legislation (statutory instrument (SI) or 'rules') is the name given to legislation which gives effect to an Act of Parliament. For example, an Act might invest powers in a body to 'set standards for education'. The secondary legislation might spell out what those educational standards are in detail. Secondary legislation is comparatively easier and quicker to change than primary legislation.

## SIGN guidelines

This acronym stands for Scottish Intercollegiate Guidelines Network. Evidence based clinical guidelines are prepared by authoritative groups on focused areas of care, such as colorectal cancer. The wide collection forms the basis of clinical standards used in healthcare in Scotland.

## ▒ Skin Care Campaign

The Skin Care Campaign is a network of voluntary health organisations and professionals concerned with skin disease. It provides information and advice on all aspects of dermatology services. ✉ ☏ 🗎 🖰

## Specialist practitioner

This term is used by nurses to describe those with additional skills and knowledge gained after registration, usually after following a specific programme of preparation approved by one of the National Boards for Nursing, Midwifery and Health Visiting. The criteria are likely to be revised in the light of the current work being undertaken by the UKCC on higher level practice.

## Standards in public life

Standards in public life are described in the seven principles that were established by the committee under the chairmanship of Lord Nolan (HMSO 1995). These principles apply to all aspects of public life. The Nolan committee set them out for the benefit of all those who serve the public in any way.

The principles are:

1. *Selflessness*: Holders of public office should take decisions solely in terms of the public interest. They should not do so in order to gain financial or other material benefits for themselves, their family or their friends.
2. *Integrity*: Holders of public office should not place themselves under any financial or other obligation to outside individuals or organisations that might influence them in the performance of their official duties.
3. *Objectivity*: In carrying out public business, including making public appointments, awarding contracts or recommending individuals for rewards and benefits, holders of public office should make choices on merit.
4. *Accountability*: Holders of public office are accountable for their decisions and actions to the public and must submit themselves to whatever scrutiny is appropriate to their office.
5. *Openness*: Holders of public office should be as open as possible about all the decisions and actions that they take. They should give reasons for their decisions and restrict information only when the public interest clearly demands it.
6. *Honesty*: Holders of public office have a duty to declare any private interests relating to their public duties and to take steps to resolve any conflicts in a way that protects the public interest.
7. *Leadership*: Holders of public office should promote and support these principles by leadership and example.

# Statutory regulatory bodies

Statutory regulatory bodies are those bodies established by law to regulate their specific professions. Each body keeps a register of its qualified practitioners and sets standards relating to entry, maintenance on and removal from its professional register. See under each individual entry for details:

- Council for the Professions Supplementary to Medicine (art/drama/music/dance therapists; chiropodists; clinical scientists in health*; dietitians; medical scientific laboratory officers; occupational therapists; paramedics*; prosthetists and orthotists; physiotherapists; orthoptists; radiographers; speech and language therapists*) (*on fast track to membership) ✉ ☏ 📄
- General Dental Council (dentists and dental technicians) ✉☏📄
- General Medical Council (doctors) ✉ ☏ 📄 🖰
- General Optical Council (opticians) ✉ ☏ 📄
- General Osteopathic Council (osteopaths) ✉ ☏ 📄
- Royal Pharmaceutical Society for Great Britain (pharmacists) ✉ ☏ 📄 @
- United Kingdom Central Council for Nursing, Midwifery and Health Visiting (nurses, midwives and health visitors) ✉ ☏ 📄 🖰.

## Strategic health authorities

The 95 health authorities (see entry) in England will be replaced in April 2002 (subject to parliamentary approval) by around 30 Strategic Health Authorities (SHAs). Many of the responsibilities previously held by Health Authorities will pass to PCTs, who will work in partnership with other bodies such as local authorities to ensure local health needs are met. SHAs will lead the strategic development of the local health service across their areas and performance manage PCTs and NHS Trusts working in those areas.

## Succession planning

Succession planning is a symbiotic relationship which fuses individuals and organisational developmental needs. It is focused on the future and the skills, knowledge and attributes that will be required within the organisation and how these can best be met. Its purpose is to develop a continuity of workforce skills that will secure the long-term stability of the organisation in delivering healthcare (Hudson 1993, Nardoni 1989).

## Underpinning philosophy

Succession planning is about valuing staff, supporting their career development needs and nurturing them to realise their maximum potential to the mutual benefit of both themselves and the current needs of the organisation. It is a responsibility that belongs to the individual as well as to the organisation (Elliot & Pickering 1997). These principles are supported by the IHSM study into creative career paths (IHSM 1996). The study established that a flexible and imaginative career culture in the NHS could lead to a more cost effective use and deployment of managers, greater motivation and satisfaction for individuals and better recruitment of talented staff in the NHS (Johns et al 1994).

## Rationale

Healthcare needs to prepare itself for the new millennium so that it is in a robust position to meet the challenges ahead. Just as there will always be a continuing need to support and develop staff, the resources to do so will always be in short supply (Benton 1997). Therefore, healthcare needs to look at flexible and innovative approaches to staff development that are aimed at all levels within the organisation and have direct relevance to organisational needs.

## Background

Succession planning and career development have attracted increasing levels of attention over recent years, promoted by:

- the loss of traditional hierarchies and career routes as healthcare as a whole adopts a flatter structure
- shortage of clinicians, due in part to a reducing labour pool to recruit from and increasing competition from other employers
- healthcare reforms which are creating new opportunities for a wider clinical voice but also demanding new skills and attributes for new roles
- the changing and expanding role of healthcare professionals.

A succession planning strategy provides a coherent and pro-active approach to these issues as it requires senior staff to look at developing more creative and flexible career opportunities for healthcare professionals to address issues of recruitment and retention. It prompts the organisation to identify current and projected resource needs and to clearly identify both the role of the organisation and that of the individual in meeting their professional development needs.

## Organisational responsibilities

For a succession planning strategy to be a useful tool, the organisation needs to have established a clear articulated view of the future. Thompson (1993) suggests that it should be informed in part by a situational analysis that evaluates how well the resources of the organisation match the needs of the environment in which it currently operates and the one it envisages in 1, 3, 5, and 10 years time, with regard to skills, skill mix and role responsibilities. The question is, how is the organisation going to ensure it has the right skills to function in this anticipated 'new world', then set the scene for implementing a succession planning strategy? Such a strategy necessitates a move away from traditional hierarchical organisational systems to a matrix-type framework that respects lateral as well as vertical movement, resulting in a variety of skill sets. The result is a workforce with a greater variety of skill sets, who are better able to be the flexible and innovative practitioners needed by the health service.

## Organisational characteristics

The most successful environment for succession planning is one which supports risk taking whilst fostering learning and development. There needs to be a belief in and a commitment to the philosophy that runs throughout the organisation (Andrica 1994) and promotes a range of opportunities that facilitate the growth and development of both the individual and the organisation. However, development does not happen in a vacuum. To be meaningful it needs to be part of both a personal and an organisational development plan.

## Individual characteristics

Healthcare professionals have a responsibility to create their own learning environment and opportunities, and to access those that are available within and external to the organisation. The organisation should recognise that a significant percentage of the workforce will be in *career maintenance* mode, whereby, beyond keeping abreast of clinical developments and best practice, they are not promotion orientated. This group must be supported in their decision. However, it must be remembered that no role is static and as the demands of healthcare change, so will the professionals' roles.

Similarly, a percentage of healthcare professionals will be *career active* and motivated by the possibilities of promotion and career development opportunities. These categories are not rigid divisions and there needs to be a mechanism for people to move between the two, depending on their energy levels, abilities and commitments.

### Outcomes

The benefits of implementing a succession planning strategy are:

- improved recruitment and retention of staff
- internal 'expert skills pool' that can be drawn upon as required
- a more flexible and creative workforce
- more cost-effective and appropriate staff development
- greater level of staff satisfaction
- improved service delivery.

The benefits of outcomes such as these are very persuasive as staff shortages have been a recurring phenomenon in healthcare (Buchan & O'May 1998). One way of helping to rewrite the script for the 21st century would be to implement a robust, high quality workforce capable of delivering the modern and dependable health service envisaged by the government (NHSE 1998b).

## Support workers

Support workers to qualified/registered healthcare professionals form an integral and vital part of the health services. They have various titles, for example, healthcare assistants, helpers or auxiliaries. They may have undertaken some form of on-the-job training, often through a National or Scottish Vocational Qualification (NVQ, SVQ). A major issue for debate is whether they should be regulated, as currently anyone can call them-selves a healthcare assistant regardless of qualifications or background. No central register exists which allows potential employers – individual or corporate – to check their competence in any way. This poses a problem when individuals, for example, are sacked for incompetence or misbehaviour, as there is little to prevent them from obtaining another post in a health setting. Some statutory regulatory bodies have a remit both for those who are professionally qualified in their field and for those who assist them. However, this is not the case in nursing and mid-wifery, the largest employers of such helpers.

## Supporting students see Clinical supervision, Mentoring, Preceptorship

S

## Teaching nursing homes

A comparatively new idea, the concept of teaching nursing homes has grown from the loss of teaching, learning and research opportunities for clinical staff, as a result of the move of much of continuing care from hospitals to the nursing home sector. The idea is based on the model of teaching hospitals and would offer all the normal facilities associated with nursing homes, but with an emphasis on building up a centre of excellence with teaching, learning, research and a range of professional development opportunities (McCormack 1999). Although the concept of teaching nursing homes is in its infancy in the UK and there is still a range of ethical and practical issues that will need sensitive and detailed exploration, this is a huge potential growth area. Pilot initiatives are already underway in the UK, with both NHS and private involvement.

# A–Z guide

## UK Council of Health Regulators

The UK Council of Health Regulators is a new body, proposed within the context of the National Plan for England (see National Plan). It is anticipated that this will link the existing and new health regulatory bodies. Further details were unavailable at the time of writing.

## UNISON

UNISON is the largest trade union in the UK with over 1.3 million members. All its members work in the public services, for private contractors providing public services, and in the essential utilities. They include manual and white collar staff working full or part time for local authorities, the NHS, colleges and schools, the electricity, gas and water industries, transport and the voluntary sector. Local stewards, who are volunteers, recruit new members, organise branches and assist members. Healthcare is one of six service groups which bring together members working in the same field. UNISON has a policy of proportionality which ensures that women are elected throughout the union in fair proportion to their membership. It also has self-organised groups which represent those who are likely to face discrimination at work, such as lesbians and gay men, women, black members and disabled members.

## United Kingdom Central Council for Nursing, Midwifery and Health Visiting

The United Kingdom Central Council for Nursing, Midwifery and Health Visiting (UKCC) was established by the Nurses, Midwives and Health Visitors Act 1979, which was amended by the Act of the same name in 1992 and then replaced by the 1997 Act of the same name. Its purpose is to establish and maintain standards of education and training and professional conduct for all those on its register. It maintains a professional register of over 630 000 names. Entry to the register is as a result of the satisfactory completion of an educational programme approved by a National Board for Nursing, Midwifery and Health Visiting in the UK, or by means of a qualification acquired outside the UK which may need to be supplemented by some UK experience before registration. Maintenance on the register is secured by meeting the profession's requirements for continuing professional development, PREP. The UKCC has power through its professional conduct mechanisms to remove a practitioner's name from the register, place an interim suspension upon a practitioner or offer a caution.

The UKCC Council consists of 40 elected members (7 nurses, 2 midwives and 1 health visitor from each of the 4 countries of the UK) and 20 Secretary of State appointed members. Members serve for a period of 5 years.

Following the Government's response to a review in 1999 (Port 1999), the UKCC and the National Boards are to be replaced by a new body. The principle of self-regulation was upheld and a decision was made to move towards one central standard setting body, to be called The Nurses and Midwives Council (see entry). ✉ ① 📄 ✏

## User involvement/partnership

In a world of uncertainty, there are two relatively certain things within the NHS: one is that the process of structural change will continue, and the second is that relationships with patients/users and professionals will be approached on a more equitable basis. In fact, it would be fair to say that the two developments are intertwined. The more any organisation looks at its services from the user perspective rather than the provider perspective the more the pressure for change will grow as the organisation sees itself in a different light. This can be a painful process, but it can also be hugely beneficial to both the patient and the healthcare professional, if the process is seen as partnership development.

There are three main areas where the involvement of patients is making an impact, but the processes and outcomes are different. It is therefore important, when all the buzz phrases such as patient partnership, patient involvement and patient empowerment are used, that it is clear which area is being talked about, and why engagement with patients and service users is so vital.

## The policy making process

This takes place at government, NHS Executive, Government Health Department, health authority and Trust level. Few would have a problem with the idea of more open, transparent and accountable decision-making processes. The involvement of both professionals and lay people results in policy and services better able to meet the needs of patients, especially where decision making is devolved as far as possible to those who will be affected by the implementation.

## Disease management

There are hundreds of charities and voluntary health organisations working in the health field. Many are household names and are substantial organisations in their own right. They fund services and invest significant amounts of money in medical research of one kind or another. Over the years these organisations have built up an enormous amount of information and knowledge about patients' experiences of living with disease or disability – particularly long-term problems. This expertise should be seen as complementary to, not in conflict with, clinical knowledge. It is different, based on the knowledge, experience and expertise of those living with a long-term problem – often encompassing every aspect of their lives and the lives of their families and carers. Such knowledge helps to interpret the lived experience of a disease, which may be substantially different from that perceived by the professional. For example, the social effects of a disease can be more devastating than the clinical effects and may be a contributory factor in why some people stop using medicines if, in the user's view, the side effects outweigh any minimal improvements in the condition it is intended to control.

These organisations are the ones who have frequently led the campaigns for more patient involvement. In the past, at times, they have been highly critical of service provision, but most are now engaging in developing positive problem-solving and partnership relationships.

### Patients/users in a one to one relationship with their health practitioner

Enabling patients to participate in their consultation by asking questions which will help them to understand the diagnosis, prognosis and the implications of their condition on their lifestyle, expectations and quality of life is essential. In this context the patient and clinician can agree a management programme which is realistic, clearly understood and therefore more likely to be implemented for optimum benefit. There is ample evidence that informed, participative patients taking responsibility for their own health, achieve better health outcomes than those who are merely passive recipients of care prescribed by a professional.

Professionals who wish to give practical effect to improved patient partnership will ensure that they keep an up-to-date database of local and national voluntary health organisations, make contact with them and are aware of their literature and the facilities they offer, such as training and education programmes for their members as well as for healthcare professionals. Contact with such organisations should result in more informed patients and professionals and prove of mutual benefit to all concerned in the positive management of a condition or disease. Proactive involvement of such organisations in any patient related activity – whether formal or informal processes of consultation are used – is essential in ensuring that patient partnership goes beyond lip service and results in meaningful and equal relationships.

## Voice

Following the abolition of the CHCs (see entry), VOICE – the Commission for Patient and Public Involvement in Health – is the name given to the proposed non-departmental public body which will represent to the Secretary to State and Parliament the views of patient organisations in relation to the running and planning of the NHS. There will also be local VOICE organisations – one per strategic health authority. Details were not available at the time of going to print.

## Walk-in centres

Walk-in centres were originally set up by private companies to provide instant access to those too busy to get to their GPs, in commuter areas like main line stations. The NHS version was established as part of the Government's initiative to provide more accessible healthcare in the NHS. No appointments are necessary and the opening hours are from early morning to late at night, 7 days a week. They are staffed by nurses and doctors. 19 centres were initially established in 1999.

## Welsh Assembly

The Government of Wales Act 1998 is the legislation which established the Welsh Assembly. The responsibilities relating to health which previously rested with the Welsh Office (see entry) have been moved to the National Assembly for Wales. The Health Promotion Authority for Wales and parts of the Welsh Health Common Services Agency have also become part of the Assembly. The Assembly is led by a First Secretary and under-secretaries are responsible for different government departments such as health.

## Welsh Health Common Services Agency

The Welsh Health Common Services Agency (WHCSA) is a special health authority responsible for providing a range of support services to the National Health Service in Wales and for advising the Welsh Office on National Health Service related issues. Some of its functions will pass to the Welsh Assembly.

## Welsh National Board for Nursing, Midwifery and Health Visiting

The Welsh National Board for Nursing, Midwifery and Health Visiting is a statutory body responsible for approving and monitoring education for nurses, midwives and health visitors in Wales, established by the Nurses, Midwives and Health Visitors Act 1979. It currently has 10 members, 7 executive and 3 non-executive. Following a government review in 1998 the Boards and the UKCC are to be replaced by a new UK statutory body to be called the Nurses and Midwives Council. The nature of representation in Wales was under discussion at the time of writing. ✉ ◑ 🖹

## 🗺 Welsh Office Health Department

The Welsh Office Health Department was responsible for strategic management, organisation development and personnel, finance, NHS Trusts and health services, primary health care and public health in respect of the management of the NHS in Wales. The Department had 6 divisions:

- Health Commissioning
- Health Services
- Health Management
- Health Financial Management
- Primary and Community Health and
- Public Health.

## White Papers

A White Paper is a government report giving information or proposals on an issue. They are sometimes, but not necessarily, preceded by a Green Paper containing proposals for discussion and consultation. White Papers can be issued by any of the four government departments in the UK. Proposals or policy changes are usually country specific and assumptions should not be made about the policy implications of any one particular White Paper across the four countries of the UK: for example, an English White Paper will not apply to Scotland.

## Workforce planning

Until the early 1990s, workforce planning had been centrally controlled with plans for clinical staff being identified at hospital level: that is, the number of clinical staff required to enter training as doctors, nurses, midwives and professions allied to medicine. The numbers were coordinated at regional health

W

authority level and passed to the Department of Health. There were always significant differences across regions, for example, London had much higher numbers because of the high ratio of teaching hospitals and an understanding that they exported these staff across the UK on completion of their training.

Project 2000 brought the integration of Schools of Nursing and Midwifery into universities, and the necessity to agree contracts for numbers to be trained arose locally between hospitals and community Trusts within the appropriate local providers of education in Higher and Further Education institutions. This could not be done on a single Trust basis as it would not be economically viable and there were insufficient experienced workforce planners and human resources experts in this field to do the work at a satisfactory level. To overcome these difficulties *education consortia* were formed. These groups are usually chaired by a chief executive of an NHS Trust and would have representatives from a Trust, social services, the independent sector and primary care, along with others relevant to the agreed geographical patch. Their purpose is to establish the workforce required in the next 3–5 years and to consider which educational institution could meet their requirements at the best value for money.

The consortia have the support of a local manager but the Regional Executive Officers have a strong supportive and, if necessary, directive input to ensure that across a region, adequate staff are coming into the system. The strength of the consortia is growing as this expertise in workforce planning and negotiations with Higher and Further Education has progressed, and as the ownership of the process becomes embedded.

## Working time regulations

These regulations are a form of European Union legislation, which came into force on 1 October 1998, limiting the number of hours worked by individuals to 48 per week. Until they are reviewed in 2003, workers in the UK can opt out of the requirements but cannot be forced to do so. Other elements include:

- shifts at night are limited to 8 hours
- staff health assessments must be undertaken
- 11 consecutive hours between each working day

- an uninterrupted rest period of not less than 24 hours in each 7 day period must be taken (this can be averaged out over a 2-week period)
- paid annual leave of at least 3 weeks, rising to 4.

Further information is available from the DTI.

## World Health Organisation

The World Health Organisation (WHO) was established in 1948 and is an international non-governmental organisation with a wide range of functions. It is mainly concerned with the promotion of cooperation in strengthening health and healthcare worldwide. Its key objective is to achieve the attainment by all peoples of the highest possible levels of health. It acts as the central authority directing international health work and establishes relationships with professional groups and government health authorities on that basis. Its functions are wide and varied. For example, it supports, on request from member states, programmes to promote health, prevent disease, train health workers best suited to local needs and strengthen national health systems. Aid is also provided in emergencies and natural disasters. It also supports global programmes of collaborative research, undertakes surveillance of communicable and non-communicable diseases and collects and disseminates health data.

W

# References

Andrica D 1994 Executive development – management succession: who will replace you? Nursing Economics (May/June) 12(3):170

Antonovsky A 1996 The salutogenic model as theory to guide health promotion. Health Promotion International 11(1):11–18

Beauchamp T L, Childress J F 1994 Principles of biomedical ethics, 4th edn. Oxford University Press, Oxford

Benton D 1997 Workforce planning. Nursing Management Feb 4(9):12–13

Buchan J, O'May F 1998 Nursing supply and demand: reviewing the evidence. Nursing Times July 1, 9(26)

Carson D, Montgomery J 1989 Nursing and the law. Macmillan, Basingstoke

Clutterbuck D 1997 Everyone needs a mentor. London Institute of Personal Development, London

Cumberlege J 1986 Neighbourhood nursing: a focus for care (The Cumberlege Report). DHSS, London

Department of Health 1983 NHS management enquiry (The Griffiths Report). DHSS, London

Department of Health 1989 Report of the advisory group in nurse prescribing (The Crown Report 1). DOH, London

Department of Health 1990 Access to Health Records Act 1990: a guide for the NHS. DOH, London

Department of Health 1997 The new NHS: modern, dependable. Cm 3807, TSO

Department of Health 1998a A first class service: quality in the new NHS. DOH, London

Department of Health 1998b Modernising health and social services. National priorities guidance 1999/00–2001/02. DOH, London

Department of Health 1998c Electronic health records options – a discussion paper. DOH, London (http://www.doh.gov.uk/nhsexipu/whatnew/ehrdis.htm)

Department of Health 1998c Better services for vulnerable people – maintaining the momentum. DOH, London

Department of Health 1999a Review of prescribing, supply and administration of medicines: final report (The Crown Report 2). DOH, London

Department of Health 1999b Information management. Making a difference: strengthening the nursing, midwifery and health visiting contribution to health and healthcare (HSG 1999/053). DOH, London

Douglas M 1992 Risk and blame. Routledge, London

Downie R S 1990 Ethics in health education: an introduction. In: Doxiadis S (ed) Ethics in health education. John Wiley, Chichester

Downie R S, Fyfe C, Tannahill A 1990 Health promotion models and values. Oxford University Press, Oxford

Edwards S D 1996 Nursing ethics – a principle-based approach. Macmillan, London

Elliott P, Pickering S 1997 The purpose of PREP. Nursing Management (June) 4(3):12–13

Exley M 1993 Building the empowered organisation. Empowerment in Organisations 1(2):4–9

Fletcher J 1966 Situation ethics SCM Press, London

Gibson C H 1991 A concept of empowerment. Journal of Advanced Nursing 16:354–356

Gilligan C 1982 In a different voice. Harvard University Press, Cambridge, MASS

Handy C 1995 Beyond certainty. Hutchinson, London

Hay J 1997 Transformational mentoring: creating developmental alliances for changing cultures. McGraw-Hill Book Company, New York

Henderson V 1966 The nature of nursing: a definition and implication for practice, research and education. Macmillan, New York

HMSO 1995 Standards in public life: the first report on the committee on standards in public life (The Nolan Report). HMSO, London

HMSO 1995 The nurses', midwives' and health visitors' (periodic registration) amendment rules approval order (The PREP Rules). Statutory Instrument 967. HMSO, London

Hokanson Hawkes J 1992 Empowerment in nursing education: concept analysis an application to philosophy, learning and instruction. Journal of Advanced Nursing 609–618

Hopson B, Scally M 1981 Life skills teaching. McGraw Hill, London

Hudson T 1993 Smart move: CEOs say succession planning up. Hospital 42

Hull C, Redfern L 1996 Profiles and portfolios. Macmillan, London

IHSM 1996 Creative career paths in the NHS. Summary of findings. NHSE, London

Johns C et al 1994 Succession management: a model for developing nurse leaders. Nursing Management USA 25(6):50–55

Johnstone M-J 1994 After virtue: a study in moral theory. Duckworth, London

Kuhn T 1970 The structure of scientific revolutions. University of Chicago Press, Chicago

Lockett T 1997 Traces of evidence. Healthcare Today 16

McCormack B 1999 Teaching nursing homes. Nursing Times, NT Nursing Homes supplement (October) 1(3):22–23

Manthey M, Miller D 1994 Empowerment through levels of authority. Journal of Nursing Administration 24(7/8):23

Nardoni R 1989 Successful succession planning. Personnel Journal May 1989 106–110

NBS 1999 Preceptorship in action. NBS, Edinburgh

NHSE 1998a Information for health. An information strategy for the modern NHS 1998–2005. DOH, Leeds

NHSE 1998b Working together – securing a quality workforce in the NHS. Department of Health, Wetherby

NHSE 1999 Code of practice on openness in the NHS. NHSE, Leeds .

NHSE 2000 Creating a 21$^{st}$ century NHS – the national plan for the new NHS. NHSE, Leeds

Noddings N 1984 Caring: a feminist approach to ethics and moral education. University of California Press, London

Parliament 1977 The NHS Act

Parliament 1997 The Government of Wales Act

Parliament 1998 The Scotland Act

Parliament 1999 The Health Act

Parliament 1999 The Public Disclosure Act

Parliament 2000 The Care Standards Bill

Port J 1999 The regulation of nurses, midwives and health visitors: report on a review of the Nurses, Midwives and Health Visitors Act 1997 (The Port Report). JM Consulting, Bristol

RPSGB 1997 Medicines, ethics and practice: guide to pharmacists. RPSGB, London

Schon D 1987 Educating the reflective practitioner. Jossey Bass, London

Scottish Executive 1998 Working together for a healthier Scotland. Scottish Executive, Edinburgh

Scottish Executive NHS MEL 1999 Managed clinical networks. Scottish Executive, Edinburgh, 10 par 3(26)

Scottish Executive 1999 Towards a healthier Scotland. A White Paper on health. Scottish Executive, Edinburgh

Scottish Executive 2000 Working together to build a healthy, caring Scotland. Scottish Executive, Edinburgh

Scottish Office 1998 Designed to care: renewing the National Health Service in Scotland. (Cmnd 3811) Edinburgh Stationery Office, Edinburgh

Seedhouse D 1986 Health: the foundations for achievement. John Wiley, Chichester

Slevin O 1999 The nurse–patient relationship: caring in a health context. In: Long A (ed) Interaction for practice in community nursing. Macmillan, London

Smith K 1999 The Gatehouse Assessment Centre integrated care pathways. Warrington Community Healthcare NHS Trust

Thompson J 1993 Strategic management – awareness and change, 2nd edn. Chapman and Hall, London

UKCC 1992 The code of professional conduct. UKCC, London

UKCC 1995 The Council's position concerning a period of support and preceptorship. Registrar's Letter 3. UKCC, London

UKCC 1998a Midwives code of practice. UKCC, London

UKCC 1998b Guidelines for records and record keeping. UKCC, London

UKCC 1999 Fitness for practice. The UKCC Commission for Nursing and Midwifery Education (The Peach Report). UKCC, London

Wallace M J 1999 Lifelong learning: PREP in action. Churchill Livingstone, Edinburgh

Walshe K 1999 You ain't seen nothing yet. HSJ 6 May 1999

Walshe K, Ham C 1997 Acting on the evidence, progress in the NHS. NHS Confederation and University of Birmingham Health Services Management Centre, Birmingham

Weisinger H 2000 Emotional intelligence at work – the untapped edge for success. Jossey Bass, San Francisco, pp xviii–xviii (Paperback edition)

Weller B (ed) 2000 Baillières nurses dictionary, 23rd edn. Baillière Tindall, London

Welsh Office 1998 NHS Wales: putting patients first. (Cmnd 3841) London Stationery Office, London

World Health Organisation 1946 Constitution. WHO, New York

World Health Organisation 1984 Report of the working group on concepts and principles of health promotion. World Health Organisation, Copenhagen

# Useful addresses/contacts

## Action for Sick Children
✉ First Floor
300 Kingston Road
London
SW20 8LX
☎ 020 8542 4848
🖰 www.actionforsickchildren.
org

## Action for Smoking and Health (ASH)
✉ 102 Clifton Street
London
EC2A 4HW
☎ 020 7739 5902
🖰 www.ash.org.uk

## Action for Victims of Medical Accidents
✉ 44 High Street
Croydon
CR0 1YB
☎ 020 8686 8333
🖷 020 8667 9065
@ admin@avma.org.uk
🖰 www.avma.org.uk

## Age Concern England
✉ Astral House
1268 London Road
London
SW16 4ER
☎ 020 8765 7200
🖰 www.ace.org.uk

## Alcoholics Anonymous (AA)
✉ PO Box 1
Stonebow House
Stonebow
York
Y01 2NJ
☎ 01904 644 026
🖰 www.alcoholics-
anonymous.org.uk

## Alzheimer's Society
✉ Gordon House
10 Greencoat Place
London
SW1P 1PH
☎ 020 7306 0606
🖰 www.alzheimers.org.uk

## American Nurses Association, Inc.
✉ 600 Maryland Avenue SW
Suite 100 West
Washington
DC 20024
☎ 202/651-7000
🖰 www.ana.org

### Arthritis Care
✉ 18 Stephenson Way
London
NW1 2HD
☎ 020 7380 6500
🖱 www.arthritiscare.org.uk

### Arthritis Research Campaign
✉ St Mary's Court
St Mary's Gate
Chesterfield
S41 7TD
Derbyshire
☎ 01256 558 033
🖱 www.arc.org.uk

### Association for All Speech-Impaired Children (AFASIC)
✉ 69–85 Old Street
London
EC1V 9HX
☎ 020 7841 8900
🖱 www.afasic.org.uk

### Association of Breast Feeding Mothers
✉ PO Box 441
St Albans
Hertfordshire
AL4 0AS
☎ 020 7813 1481

### Association of Community Health Councils (England and Wales)
✉ 30 Drayton Park
London
N5 1PB
☎ 020 7609 8405

📄 020 7700 1152
🖱 www.achced.org.uk

### Association of Healthcare Human Resource Management
✉ AHHRM c/o NHSP
King Square House
Bristol
BS2 8EE
🖱 www.ahhrm.org.uk

### Association of Medical Research Charities
✉ 29–35 Farringdon Road
London
EC1M 3JF
☎ 020 7404 6454
📄 020 7404 6448
@ info@amrc.org.uk

### Association of Medical Secretaries, Practice Managers, Administrators and Receptionists (AMSPAR)
✉ Tavistock House North
Tavistock Square
London
WC1H 9LN
☎ 020 7387 6005
🖱 www.amspar.co.uk

### Association of Radical Midwives
✉ 62 Greetby Hill
Ormskirk
Lancashire
L39 2DT
☎ 01695 572776
🖱 www.radmid.demon.co.uk

**Association for Spina Bifida and Hydrocephalus (ASBAH)**
✉ 42 Park Road
Peterborough
PE1 2UQ
☎ 01733 555988
🖰 www.asbah.org

**Association for Spinal Injury Research, Rehabilitation and Reintegration (ASPIRE)**
✉ Royal National
Orthopaedic Hospital
Brokley Hill
Stanmore
Middlesex
HA7 4LP
☎ 020 8954 0701
🖰 www.aspire.org.uk

**Audit Commission**
✉ 1 Vincent Square
London
SW12 2PN
🖰 www.audit-com.gov.uk

**Australian Nursing Federation**
✉ Unit 3
28 Eyre Street
Kingston
ACT 2604
☎ 61 2 6232 6533
🖰 www.anf.org.au

**Baby Life Support Systems (BLISS)**
✉ 2nd Floor
Camelford House
87–89 Albert Embankment
London
SE1 7TP
☎ 020 7820 9471
🖰 www.bliss.org.uk

**The Baby Network**
✉ c/o BLISS
2nd Floor
Camelford House
87–89 Albert Embankment
London
SE1 7TP
☎ 020 7820 9471
🖺 020 7820 9567
@ suzannedobson@bliss.org.uk

**BackCare**
@ back-pain@compuserve.com
🖰 www.backpain.org

**Breast Cancer Care**
✉ Kiln House
210 New Kings Road
London
SW6 4NZ
☎ 020 7384 2984
🖰 www.breastcancercare.org.uk

**British Agencies for Adoption and Fostering**
✉ Skyline House
200 Union Street
London
SE1 0LX
☎ 020 7593 2000
🖰 www.baaf.org.uk

**British Association for Cancer United Patients (BACUP)**
✉ 3 Bath Place
Rivington Street
London
EC2A 3JR
☎ 020 7696 9003
🖱 www.cancerbacup.org.uk

**British Association for Counselling (BAC)**
✉ 1 Regent Place
Rugby
Warwickshire
CV21 2PJ
☎ 0870 443 5252
📄 0870 443 5160
@ bac@bac.co.uk
🖱 www.counselling.co.uk

**The British Association of Occupational Therapists/ College of Occupational Therapists**
✉ 106–114 Borough High Street
Southwark
London
SE1 1LB
☎ 020 7357 6480
📄 020 7450 2249
🖱 www.baot.co.uk

**British Colostomy Association**
✉ 15 Station Road
Reading
Berkshire
RG1 1LG
☎ 0118 939 153
🖱 www.bcass.org.uk

**British Complementary Medicine Association (BCMA)**
✉ Kensington House
33 Imperial Square
Cheltenham
Gloucester
GL50 1QZ
☎ 01242 519 911
🖱 www.bcma.co.uk

**British Deaf Association**
✉ 1–3 Worship Street
London
EC2A 2AB
☎ 020 7588 3520
🖱 www.bda.org.uk

**British Dental Association**
✉ 64 Wimpole Street
London
W1M 8AL
☎ 020 7935 0875
🖱 www.bda-dentistry.org.uk

**The British Dietetic Association**
✉ 5th Floor
Elizabeth House
22 Suffolk Street
Queensway
Birmingham
B1 1LS
☎ 0121 616 4913
📄 0121 616 4901
🖱 www.bda.uk.com

## British Epilepsy Association

✉ Anstey House
Gate Way Drive
Yeadon
Leeds
LS19 7XY
☎ 0113 210 8800
🖱 www.epilepsy.org.uk

## British Geriatrics Society (BGS)

✉ 31 St John's Square
London
EC1M 4DN
☎ 020 7608 1369
🖱 www.bgs.org.uk

## British Heart Foundation

✉ 14 Fitzhardinge Street
London
W1H 4DH
☎ 020 7935 0185
🖨 020 7486 5820
🖱 www.bhf.org.uk

## British Homeopathic Association

✉ 15 Clerkenwell Close
London
EC1R 0AA
☎ 020 7566 7800
🖱 www.trusthomeopathy.org

## British Institute for Brain Injured Children (BIBIC)

✉ Knowle Hall
Bridgewater
Somerset
TA7 8PJ
☎ 01278 684 060
🖱 www.bibic.org.uk

## British Institute of Radiology

✉ 36 Portland Place
London
W1N 4AT
☎ 020 7307 1400
🖱 www.bir.org.uk

## British Kidney Patient Association (BKPA)

✉ Bordon
Hampshire
GU35 9JZ
☎ 01402 472 021

## British Lung Foundation

✉ 78 Hatton Garden
London
EC1N 8LD
☎ 020 7831 5831
🖨 020 7831 5832
@ bif_user@gpiag-asthma.org
🖱 www.lunguk.org

## British Medical Association (BMA)

✉ BMA House
Tavistock Square
London
WC1H 9JP
☎ 020 7388 8296
🖱 www.bma.org.uk

## The British Nutrition Foundation

✉ High Holborn House
52–54 High Holborn

London
WC1V 6RQ
☎ 020 7404 6504
📄 020 7404 6747
@ postbox@nutrition.org.uk

## British Organ Donor Society (BODY)

✉ Balsham
Cambridge
CB1 6DL
☎ 01223 893636
🖱 www.argonet.co.uk/body/

## British Pregnancy Advisory Service (BPAS)

✉ Austy Manor Woottom
Wawen
Solihull
West Midlands
B95 6BX
☎ 01564 793 225
🖱 www.bpas.org

## British Psychological Society

✉ St Andrews House
48 Princess Road East
Leicester
LE1 7DR
☎ 01162 549568
📄 01162 470787

## British Red Cross Society (BRCS)

✉ 9 Grosvenor Crescent
London
SW1X 7EJ
☎ 020 7235 5454
🖱 www.redcross.org.uk

## British United Provident Association (BUPA)

✉ BUPA House
15–19 Bloomsbury Way
London
WC1A 2BA
☎ 020 7656 2000
🖱 www.bupa.co.uk

## Brittle Bone Society

✉ 30 Guthrie Street
Dundee
DD1 5BS
☎ 01382 204 446
🖱 www.brittlebone.org

## Brook Advisory Centres

✉ Studio 421
Highgate Studios
51–79 Highgate Road
London
NW5 1TL
☎ 020 7284 6070
🖱 www.brookcentres.org.uk

## Canadian Nurses' Association

✉ 50 Driveway
Ottawa
Ontario
K2P 1E2
☎ 613 237 2133
🖱 www.cna-nurses.ca

## CancerBACUP

✉ 3 Bath Place
Rivington Street
London
EC2A 3DR
☎ 020 7920 7233

Freephone helpline: 0808 800 1234

📄 020 7696 9002

@ jbrodie@cancerbacup.org

🖰 www.cancerbacup.org.uk

## Cancerlink

✉ 11–21 Northdown Street
London
N1 9NB

☎ 020 7833 2818

📄 020 7833 4963

@ cancerlink@cancerlink.
org.uk

🖰 www.cancerlink.org

## Carers National Association

✉ Ruth Pitter House
20–25 Glasshouse Yard
London
EC1A 4JT

☎ 020 7490 8818

@ martin@ukcarers.org

🖰 www.carersnorth.demon.
co.uk

## Centre for Policy on Ageing

✉ 19–23 Ironmonger Row
London
EC1V 3QP

☎ 020 7253 1787

🖰 www.cpa.org.uk

## Chartered Society of Physiotherapy

✉ 14 Bedford Row
London
WC1R 4ED

☎ 020 7306 6666

📄 020 7306 6661

🖰 www.csphysio.org.uk

## Childline

✉ 2nd Floor
Royal Mail Buildings
Studd Street
London
N1 0QW

☎ 020 7329 1000

🖰 www.childline.org.uk

## Clare Maxwell Hudson School of Massage

✉ Lower Ground Floor
York Street Chambers
68–72 York Street
London
W1H 1DF

☎ 020 7724 7198

🖰 www.cmhmassage.co.uk

## Clinical Standards Board for Scotland

✉ Elliott House
8–10 Hillside Crescent
Edinburgh
EH7 5EA

☎ 0131 623 4300

📄 0131 623 4299

@ comments@
clinicalstandards.org

## Coeliac Society of the United Kingdom

✉ PO Box 220
High Wycombe
Buckinghamshire
HP11 2HY

☎ 01494 437 298

🖰 www.coeliac.co.uk

**College of Health**
✉ St Margaret's House
21 Old Ford Street
London
E2 9PL
@ info@tcoh.demon.co.uk

**College of Occupational Therapists**
✉ 104–114 Borough High Street
Southwark
London
SE1 1LB
☎ 020 7357 6480
🖰 www.cot.co.uk

**College of Radiologists**
✉ 38 Portland Place
London
W1N 4JQ
☎ 020 7636 4432
🖹 020 7323 3100
@ enquiries@rcr.ac.uk

**College of Speech and Language Therapists**
✉ 2 White Hart Yard
London
SE1 1MX
🖰 www.RCSLT.org

**Commission for Racial Equality**
✉ Elliot House
10–12 Allington Street
London
SW1E 5EH
☎ 020 7828 7022
🖰 www.cre.gov.uk

**Community and District Nursing Association (CDNA)**
✉ Westel House
32–38 Uxbridge Road
Ealing
London
W5 2BS
☎ 020 8280 5342
🖰 http://www.edna.tvu.ac.uk

**Community Drug Project (CDP)**
✉ 9a Brockley Cross
Brockley
London
SE4 2AB
☎ 020 7582 2200
🖰 www.communitydrug-project.org

**Community Hospitals Association**
✉ Meadow Brow
Broadway Road
Ilminster
Somerset
TA19 9RG
☎ 01460 55951
🖹 01460 53207
@ commhosp@globalnet.co.uk
🖰 www.users.globalnet.co.uk/-commhosp

**Community Practitioners' and Health Visitors' Association (CPHVA)**
✉ 40 Bermondsey Street
London
SE1 3UD

☎ 020 7939 7000
🖹 020 7403 2976
🖰 www.msfcphva.org

## Confederation of Healing Organisations
✉ The Red and White House
113 High Street
Berkhamstead
Hertfordshire
HP4 2DJ
☎ 01442 870 660
🖰 http://drive.to/cho

## Consumer Health Information Centre
✉ PAGB
Vernon House
Sicilian Avenue
London
WC1A 2QH
☎ 020 7421 9319
🖹 020 7421 9317
@ karen.kelshaw@pagb.co.uk
🖰 www.chic.org.uk

## Contact a Family
✉ 170 Tottenham Court Road
London
W1P 0HA
☎ 020 7383 3555
🖹 020 7383 0259
@ info@cafamily.org.uk
🖰 www.cafamily.org.uk

## Coronary Prevention Group (CPG)
✉ 2 Taviton Street

London
WC1H 0BT
☎ 020 7927 2125
🖰 www.healthnet.org.uk

## Council for Complementary and Alternative Medicines
✉ Park House
206–208 Latimer Road
London
W10 6RE
☎ 0181 968 3862
🖹 0181 968 3469

## Council for the Professions Supplementary to Medicine (CPSM)
✉ Park House
184 Kennington Park Road
London
SE11 4BU
☎ 020 7582 0866
🖹 020 7820 9684

## Cruse Bereavement Care
✉ Cruse House
126 Sheen Road
Richmond
Surrey
TW9 1UR
☎ 020 8940 4818
🖰 www.crusebereavement-care.org.uk

## Cystic Fibrosis Trust
✉ 11 London Road
Bromley
Kent
BR1 1BY

① 020 8464 7211
⌇ www.cftrust.org.uk

**Department of Health**
✉ Richmond House
79 Whitehall
London
SW1A 2NS
① 020 7210 4850
⌇ www.doh.gov.uk

**Department for International Development**
✉ 94 Victoria Street
London
SW1E 5JL
① 020 7917 0503/0304

**Department of Health and Social Services, Northern Ireland**
✉ Castle Buildings
Upper Newtownards Road
Belfast
BT4 3SF
① 01232 520520

**Department of Social Security**
✉ Richmond House
79 Whitehall
London
SW1A 2NS
① 020 7210 3000
⌇ www.dss.gov.uk

**Depressives Anonymous (Fellowship of)**
✉ 57 Moira Court
Trinity Court

London
SW 17
① 020 8767 1920

**Diabetes Help (National)**
✉ 177a Tennison Road
London
SE25 5NF
① 020 8656 5467

**Diabetes UK**
✉ 10 Queen Anne Street
London
W1G 9LH
① 020 7323 1531
⌇ www.diabetes.org.uk

**Disabled Living Foundation**
✉ 380–384 Harrow Road
London
W9 3HU
① 020 7289 6111
⌇ www.dlf.org.uk

**Disablement Information and Advice Lines (DIAL UK)**
✉ St Catherines
Tickhill Road
Doncaster
DN4 8QN
① 01302 310 123
⌇ www.members.aol.com/dialuk

**Down's Syndrome Association**
✉ 155 Mitcham Road
London

SW17 9PG
① 020 8682 4001
⌐ www.downs-syndrome.
org.uk

**English National Board for
Nursing, Midwifery and
Health Visiting**
✉ Victory House
170 Tottenham Court Road
London
W1P 0HA
① 020 7388 3131
▤ 020 7383 4031
⌐ www.enb.org.uk

**Equal Opportunities
Commission (EOC)**
✉ Arndale House
Arndale Centre
Manchester
M4 3EQ
① 0161 833 9244
@ info@eoc.org.uk
⌐ www.eoc.org.uk

**Family Planning Association
(fpa)**
*England*
✉ 2-12 Pentonville Road
London
N1 9PF
① 020 7254 6251
⌐ www.fpa.org.uk
*Wales*
✉ Ground Floor
Riverside House
31 Cathedral Road
Cardiff
CF11 9HB

*Northern Ireland*
✉ 113 University Street
Belfast
BT7 1HP
*Scotland*
✉ Unit 10
Firhill Business Centre
Firhill Road
Glasgow
G20 7BA
⌐ www.fpa.org.uk

**Family Welfare
Association**
✉ 501-505 Kingland Road
London
E8 4AU
① 020 7254 6251

**Foundation for the Study of
Infant Deaths**
✉ Artillery House
11-19 Artillery Row
London
SW1P 1RT
① 020 7222 8001
⌐ www.sids.org.uk

**Gamblers Anonymous and
Gam-Anon**
✉ PO Box 88
London
SW10 0EO
① 020 7384 3040

**General Dental Council**
✉ 37 Wimpole Street
London
WIM 8DQ
① 020 7887 3800
▤ 020 7224 3294

**General Medical Council (GMC)**
✉ 178 Great Portland Street
London
W1N 3XX
☎ 020 7580 7642
🖷 020 7915 3641
🖰 www.gmc-uk.org

**General Optical Council**
✉ 41 Harley Street
London
W1N 2DJ
☎ 020 7580 3898
🖷 020 7436 3525

**General Osteopathic Council**
✉ Osteopathy House
176 Tower Bridge Road
London
SE1 3LU
☎/🖷 020 7357 6655

**Genetic Interest Group**
✉ Unit 4D
Leroy House
436 Essex Road
London
N1 3QP
☎ 020 7704 3141
🖷 020 7359 1447
@ mail@gig.org.uk
🖰 www.gig.org.uk

**Gingerbread (Association for One Parent Families)**
✉ 16–17 Clerkenwell Close
London
EC1A 0AN
☎ 020 7366 8183
🖰 www.gingerbread.org.uk

**Guillain-Barré Syndrome Support Group**
✉ LCC Offices
Eastgate
Sleaford
Lincolnshire
NG34 7EB
☎ 0800 374803
🖰 www.gbs.org.uk

**Haemophilia Society**
✉ Chesterfield House
385 Euston Road
London
NW1 3AU
☎ 020 7380 0600
🖰 www.haemophilia.org.uk

**Health Advisory Service**
✉ HAS 2000
11 Grosvenor Crescent
London
SW1X 7EE
☎ 020 7838 9944
🖷 020 7245 042

**Health Coalition Initiative**
✉ 28 Queensbury Street
London
N1 3AD
☎ 020 7688 9208
🖷 020 7359 4583
@ tinafunnell@compuserve.com

**Health Development Agency**
✉ Trevelyan House

30 Great Peter Street
London
SW1P 2HW
℡ 020 7222 5300
🖰 www.hea.org.uk

## Health Education Authority
✉ Trevelyan House
30 Great Peter Street
London
SW1 2HW
℡ 020 7222 5300

## Health Education Board for Scotland (HEBS)
✉ Research and Evaluation
Division
Health Education Board for
Scotland
Woodburn House
Canaan Lane
Edinburgh
EH10 4SG
℡ 0131 536 5500 (HEBS
Switchboard)
℡ 0131 536 5588 (Divisional
Secretary)

## Health Promotion Authority for Wales
✉ Health Promotion Wales
Ffynnon-las
Ty Glas Avenue
Llanishen
Cardiff
CF4 5DZ

## Health and Safety Executive
✉ Rose Court
2 Southwark Bridge

London
SE1 9HS
℡ 020 7717 6000
🖰 www.hse.gov.uk

## Health Service Careers
✉ PO Box 204
London
SE99 7UW

## Health Service Commissioner
✉ 13th Floor Millbank
Millbank Tower
London
SW1P 4QP
℡ 0845 0154033
🖰 www.health.ombudsman.
org.uk

## Health Service Ombudsman
✉ Millbank Tower
Millbank
London
SW1P 4QP
℡ 020 7717 4051
🖹 020 7217 4000
🖰 www.ombudsman.org.uk

## Help the Aged
✉ St James's Walk
Clerkenwell Green
London
EC1R 0BE
℡ 020 7253 0253
🖰 www.helptheaged.org.uk

## Herpes Association
✉ 41 North Road
London

N7 9DP
☎ 020 7609 9061

## Hospice Information Service

✉ St Christopher's Hospice
51–59 Lawrie Park Road
Sydenham
London
SE26 6DZ
☎ 020 8778 9252
🖰 www.hospiceinformation.
co.uk

## Huntingdon's Disease Association

✉ 108 Battersea High Street
London
SW11 3HP
☎ 020 7223 7000
🖰 www.had.org.uk

## Hysterectomy Association

✉ 51 Burton Road
Coton-in-the-Elms
Derbyshire
DE12 8HJ
☎ 01283 763446
🖰 www.hysterectomy-
association.org.uk

## Ileostomy and Internal Pouch Support Group

✉ PO Box 132
Scunthorpe
Lincolnshire
DN15 9YW
☎ 01724 720150
🖹 01724 721601
🖰 www.ileostomypouch.
demon.co.uk

## Imperial Cancer Research Fund (ICRF)

✉ 61 Lincoln's Inn Fields
London
WC2A 3PX
☎ 020 7242 0200
🖰 www.imperialcancer.co.uk

## Independent Healthcare Association (IHA)

✉ 22 Little Russell Street
London
WC1 2HT
☎ 020 7430 0537
🖹 020 7242 2681
🖰 www.iha.org.uk

## Institute of Chiropodists and Podiatrists

✉ 27 Wright Street
Southport
Merseyside
PR9 0TL
☎ 01704 546141
🖰 www.inst-chiropodist.
org.uk

## Institute of Complementary Medicine

✉ PO Box 194
London
SE16 7QZ
☎ 020 7237 5165

## Institute of Environmental Health Officers (IEHO)

✉ Chadwick Court
15 Hatfields
London
SE1 8DJ

① 020 7928 6006
🖰 www.cieh.org.uk

## International Confederation of Midwives
✉ Eisenhowerlaan 138
2517KN
The Hague
The Netherlands
① 00 1 31 70 30 60520
🖰 www.intlmidwives.org

## International Council of Nurses
✉ 3 Place Jean-Marteau
1201 Geneva
Switzerland
① 00 1 41 22 908 01 00
🖰 www.icn.ch

## International Health Exchange
✉ 134 Lower Marsh
London
SE1 7AE
① 020 7620 3333
🖰 www.ihe.org.uk

## International Voluntary Service
✉ Old Hall
East Bergholt
Colchester
CO7 6TQ
① 01206 298215
🖰 www.ivsgbn.co.uk

## Invalid Children's Aid Nationwide (ICAN)
✉ 4 Dyer's Buildings
Holborn

London
EC1N 2QP
① 0870 010 4066
🖰 www.ican.org.uk

## Irish Nurses Organisation and National Council of Nurses
✉ 11 Fitzwilliam Place
Dublin 2
Ireland
① 00 353 1676 760 137
🖰 www.ino.ie

## Jewish Bereavement Counselling Service
✉ PO Box 6748
London
N3 3BX
① 020 8349 0839

## Jewish Care
✉ Stuart Young House
221 Golders Green Road
London
NW11 9DQ
① 020 8458 3282
🖰 www.jewishcare.org

## Jewish Social Services
✉ Stuart Young House
221 Golders Green Road
London
NW11 9DQ
① 020 8458 3282

## Kidscape Campaign for Children's Safety
✉ 2 Grosvenor Gardens
London
SW1W 0DH

☎ 020 730 3300
🖱 www.kidscape.org.uk

### King Edward's Hospital Fund for London
✉ 56 Weymouth Street
London
W1G 6NX
☎ 020 7467 3920
🖱 www.kingedwardVII.com

### King's Fund
✉ 11–13 Cavendish Square
London
W1M 0AN
☎ 020 7307 2400
📄 020 7307 2801
🖱 www.kingsfund.org.uk

### Leukaemia Care Society
✉ 2 Shrubbery Avenue
Worcester
WR1 1QH
☎ 01392 464848
🖱 www.leukaemiacare.org

### Leukaemia Research Fund
✉ 43 Great Ormond Street
London
WC1N 3JJ
☎ 020 7405 0101
🖱 www.lrf.org.uk

### London College Of Massage
✉ 5–6 Newman Passage
London
W1P 3PF
☎ 020 7323 3574
🖱 www.massagelondon.com

### London Lighthouse
✉ 111–117 Lancaster Road
London
W11 1QT
☎ 020 7792 1200
🖱 www.london-lighthouse.org.uk

### Long-term Medical Conditions Alliance
✉ Unit 212
16 Baldwins Gardens
London
EC1N 7RJ
☎ 020 7813 3637
📄 020 7813 3640
@ alliance@lmca.demon.co.uk
🖱 www.lmca.demon.co.uk

### Lymphoma Association
✉ PO Box 386
Aylesbury
Bucks
HP20 2GA
☎ 0808 808 5555
🖱 www.lymphoma.org.uk

### Macmillan Cancer Relief
✉ 89 Albert Embankment
London
SE1 7UQ
☎ 020 7840 7840
🖱 www.macmillan.org.uk

### Malcolm Sargent Cancer Fund for Children
✉ Griffin House
161 Hammersmith Road
London
W6 8SG

☎ 020 8252 2800
🖹 020 8752 2806
🖰 www.sargent.org

## Marie Curie Cancer Care
✉ 89 Albert Embankment
London
SE1 7TP
☎ 020 7599 7777
🖰 www.mariecurie.org.uk

## Marie Stopes Clinic
✉ Marie Stopes House
108 Whitfield Street
London
W1P 6BE
☎ 020 7388 0662
🖰 www.mariestopes.org.uk

## Medic Alert Foundation
✉ 1 Bridge Wharf
156 Caledonian Road
London
N1 9UU
☎ 020 7833 3034
🖰 www.membership@
medicalert.org.uk

## Medical Defence Union
✉ 230 Blackfriars Road
London
SE1 8PJ
☎ 020 7200 1500
🖹 020 7202 1666
@ mdu@the-mdu.com

## Medical Research Charities
✉ 61 Gray's Inn Road
London
WC1X 8TL

☎ 020 7242 2472
🖹 020 7242 2484
@ omfp-amrc.org.uk
🖰 www.amrc.org.uk

## Medical Research Council
✉ 20 Park Crescent
London
W1N 4AL
☎ 020 7636 5422
🖰 www.mrc.ac.uk

## Medicines Control Agency
✉ 1 Nine Elms Lane
Vauxhall
London
SW8 5NQ
☎ 020 7273 0000
🖹 020 7273 0353

## Mental After Care Association
✉ 25 Bedford Square
London
WC1B 38W
☎ 020 7436 6194
🖰 www.maca.org.uk

## Mental Health Act Commission
✉ Maid Marian House
56 Hounds Gate
Nottingham
NG1 6BG
☎ 0115 943 7100
🖹 0115 943 7101

## Mental Welfare Commission
✉ K Floor
Argyle House

3 Lady Lawson Street
Edinburgh
EH3 9SH
☎ 0131 222 61111

## Midwives Information and Resource Service
✉ 9 Elmdale Road
Clifton
Bristol
BS8 1SL
☎ 01179 251791
🖰 www.midirs.org

## The Migraine Trust
✉ 45 Great Ormond Street
London
WC1N 3HD
☎ 020 7831 4818

## MIND (National Association for Mental Health)
✉ Granta House
15–19 Broadway
Stratford
London
E15 4BQ
☎ 0208 519 2122 (Office)
☎ 0208 522 1728 (Information, London)
☎ 0345 660163 (Information, outside London)
@ contact@mind.org.uk
🖰 MIND at http://www.community-care.org.uk/charity/mind/html
Information helpline:
Mindinfoline

## Mind Cymru
✉ 3rd Floor Quebec House

Castlebridge
Cowbridge Road East
Cardiff
CF11 9AB

## Minority Rights Group
✉ 379 Brixton Road
London
SW9 7DE
☎ 020 7978 9498
🖰 www.minorityrights.org

## Miscarriage Association
✉ c/o Clayton Hospital
Northgate
Wakefield
West Yorkshire
WF1 3JS
☎ 01924 200799
🖰 www.miscarriage-association.org.uk

## Motor Neurone Disease Association
✉ PO Box 246
Northampton
NN1 2PR
☎ 01604 250505
🖰 www.mndassociation.org

## MSF
✉ 33–37 Moreland Street
London
EC1V 8BB
🖰 www.msf.org.uk

## Multiple Sclerosis Society of Great Britain and Northern Ireland
✉ National Centre

372 Edgware Road
London
NW2 6ND
① 020 7610 7171
⌐ www.mssociety.org.uk

## Muscular Dystrophy Group
✉ 7–11 Prescott Place
London
SW4 6BS
① 020 7720 8055
⌐ www.mssociety.org.uk

## Myasthenia Gravis Association
✉ Keynes House
Chestes Park
Alfreton Road
Derby
DE21 4AS
① 01332 290219
⌐ www.crabby.demon.co.
uk/mga

## Narcotics Anonymous
✉ 202 City Road
London
EC1V 2PH
① 020 7251 4007
⌐ www.na.org

## National AIDS Helpline
✉ HealthwiseHelpline
Limited
1st Floor
Cavern Court
8 Matthews Street
Liverpool
LT6 RE
① 0151 227 4150

## National AIDS Trust
✉ 196 Old Street
London
EC1V 9FR
① 020 7814 6767
⌐ www.nat.org.uk

## National Assembly for Wales
✉ Crown Buildings
Cathays Park
Cardiff
CG10 1DX
① 02920 825111
⌐ www.wales.gov.uk

## National Association of Bereavement Services
✉ 2nd Floor
4 Pinchin Street
London
E1 SFA
① 020 7709 9090
⌐ Website under construction

## National Association of Carers
✉ 20–25 Glasshouse Yard
London
EC1A 4JS
① 020 7490 8818
▤ 020 7490 8824

## National Association of Citizens' Advice Bureaux
✉ 15–123 Pentonville Road
London
N1 9LZ
① 020 7833 2181
⌐ www.nacab.org.uk

**National Association for Colitis and Crohn's Disease**
✉ 4 Beaumont House
Sutton Road
St. Albans
Herts
AL1 5HH
☎ 01727 844296
🖰 www.nacc.org.uk

**National Association of Laryngectomy Clubs**
✉ Ground Floor
Rickett Street
London
SW6 1RU
☎ 020 7381 9993

**National Association of Patient Participation**
✉ 9 Lymington Road
Wallasey
Wirral
L44 3EG
☎ 0151 630 5786

**National Association for Premenstrual Syndrome**
✉ 2 East Point
High Street
Seal
Kent
TN15 0EG
☎ 01732 760011
🖰 www.pms.org.uk

**National Asthma Campaign**
✉ Providence House
Providence Place
London

N1 0NT
☎ 020 7226 2260
🖰 www.asthma.org.uk

**National Audit Office**
✉ 157 Buckingham
Palace Road
Victoria
London
SW19 5P
☎ 020 7798 7000
📄 020 7828 3774

**National Back Pain Association**
✉ 16 Elm Tree Road
Teddington
Middlesex
TW11 8ST
☎ 020 8977 5474
🖰 www.backpain.org

**National Board for Northern Ireland**
✉ Centre House
79 Chichester Street
Belfast
BT1 4JE
☎ 01232 238152
📄 01232 333298

**National Board for Scotland**
✉ 22 Queen Street
Edinburgh
EH4 1NT
☎ 0131 226 7371
📄 0131 225 9970

**National Childbirth Trust (NCT)**
✉ Alexandra House
Oldham Terrace

London
W3 6NH
✆ 0870 444 8707
🖰 www.nct-online.org

**National College of Occupational Therapists**
✉ 106–114 Borough
High Street
Southwark
London
SE1 1TB
✆ 020 7357 5480
🖨 020 7450 2299
🖰 www.cot.co.uk

**National Council for Civil Liberties**
✉ 21 Tabard Street
London
SE1 4LA
✆ 020 7403 3888
🖰 www.liberty.org.uk

**National Council for Hospice and Specialist Palliative Care Services**
✉ First Floor
34–44 Britannia Street
London
WC1X 9JG
✆ 020 7520 8299
🖨 020 7520 8298
@ enquiries@hospice-spc-council.org.uk
🖰 www.hospice-spc-council.org.uk

**National Council for One Parent Families**
✉ 255 Kentish Town Road
London

NW5 2LX
✆ 020 7428 5400
🖰 www.oneparentfamilies.org.uk

**National Council for Vocational Qualifications**
✉ 83 Piccadilly
London
W1J 8QA
✆ 020 7509 5555
🖰 www.qca.nq.uk

**National Family Mediation**
✉ 9 Tavistock Place
London
WC1H 95N
✆ 020 7383 5993
🖰 www.nfm.u-net.com/

**National Federation of Kidney Patients' Associations**
✉ 6 Stanley Street
Worksop
Notts
S81 7HX
✆ 01909 487795
🖰 www.kidney.org.uk

**National Information Forum**
✉ Post Point 10/10
BT Burne House
Bell Street
London
NW1 5BZ
✆ 020 7402 6681
🖨 020 7402 1250
🖰 www.nil.org.uk

**National Osteoporosis Society**
✉ PO Box 10
Radstock
Bath
BA3 3YB
☎ 01761 471771
🖱 www.nos.org.uk

**National Schizophrenia Fellowship (NSF)**
✉ 30 Tabernacle Street
London
EC2A 4DD
☎ 020 8974 6814 (Helpline)
☎ 020 7330 9100 (Administration)
🖷 020 7330 9102 (Administration)
@ advice@nsf.org.uk

**National Society for Epilepsy**
✉ Chalfont St Peter
Bucks
SL9 0RJ
☎ 01494 601300
🖱 www.epilepsynse.org.uk

**National Society for Mentally Handicapped People in Residential Care (RESCARE)**
✉ Rayner House
23 Higher Hillgate
Stockport
Cheshire
SK1 3ER
☎ 0161 474 7323
🖱 www.rescare.org.uk

**National Society for the Prevention of Cruelty to Children (NSPCC)**
✉ 42 Curtain Road
London
EC2A 3NH
☎ 020 7825 2500
🖱 www.nscpp.org.uk

**Neonatal Nurses Association (NNA)**
✉ 7 Milton Chambers
19 Milton Street
Nottingham
NG1 3EN
☎ 0115 941 7224

**Neurological Alliance**
✉ c/o The Multiple Sclerosis Society
The MS National Centre
372 Edgware Road
Cricklewood
London
NW2 6ND
☎ 020 8438 0700
🖷 020 8438 0877
🖱 www.mssociety.org.uk

**NHS Direct**
☎ 0845 4647 (24 hours)
🖱 www.nhsdirect.nhs.uk

**NHS Executive**
✉ Quarry House
Quarry Hill
Leeds
L52 7EU
☎ 0113 254 5000
🖱 www.open.gov.uk/doh/nhs.htm

✆ www.nhs.uk
✆ www.nhsdirect.nhs.uk

## Northern Institute of Massage
✉ 14–16 St Mary's Place
Bury
Lancs
BL9 0DZ
☎ 0161 797 1800
✆ www.nim56.co.uk

## Northern Ireland Audit Office
✉ 106 University Street
Belfast
BT7 1EU
☎ 01232 25100
🖹 01232 251051

## Nuffield Nursing Homes Trust
✉ North London Hospital
Cavell Drive
Uplands Park Road
Enfield
Middlesex
EN2 7PR
☎ 020 7266 4747

## Nurses' Fund for Nurses
✉ 2nd Floor
380 Harrow Road
London
W9 2HU
☎ 020 7266 4747
✆ Website under construction

## Nurses Welfare Service
✉ Victoria Chambers
16–18 Strutton Ground

London
SW1P 2HP
☎ 020 7222 1563
🖹 020 7799 1467

## The Office of the Information Commissioner
✉ 18 Lower Leeson Street
Dublin 2
Ireland
☎ +353 1 678 5222
🖹 +353 1 661 0570
@ foi@ombudsman.irlgov.ie

## Order of St John
✉ Priory House
25 St John's Lane
Clerkenwell
London
EC1M 4PP
☎ 020 7253 6644
✆ www.sja.org.uk

## Paget's Disease Association
✉ 323 Manchester Road
Walken
Worsley
Manchester
M28 3HH
☎ 0161 799 4646
✆ www.paget.org.uk

## Parkinson's Disease Society
✉ 215 Vauxhall Bridge Road
London
SW1V 1EJ
☎ 020 79318 080
✆ Website under construction

**Partially Sighted Society**
✉ 9 Plato Place
72-74 St Dionis Road
London
SW6 4TU
☎ 020 7371 0289

**The Patients' Association**
✉ PO Box 935
Harrow
Middlesex
HA1 3YT
☎ 020 8423 9111
☎ 0845 608 4455 (Helpline)
🖷 020 8423 9119

**The Patients' Forum**
✉ 11 John Street
London
WC1N 2EB
☎ 020 7831 6799
🖰 www.patientsforum.
org.uk

**Patient Information Forum**
✉ c/o Beki Moult
PIF Membership Secretary
Family Resource Manager
The Hospital for Sick Children
Great Ormond Street
London
WC1N 3JH

**Play Matters (National Toy Libraries Association)**
✉ 68 Churchway
London
NW1 1LT
☎ 020 7387 9592
🖰 www.charitynet.org/~natll

**Poisons Unit Medical-Toxicology**
✉ Avonley Road
London
SE14 5ER
☎ 020 7955 5095
🖰 www.medtox.org

**Pregnancy Advisory Service**
✉ 26 Bedford Square
London
WC1B 3HH
☎ 020 7637 8962
🖰 www.bpas.org

**Primary Immunodeficiency Association**
✉ Alliance House
12 Caxton Street
London
SW1H 0QS
☎ 020 7976 7640
🖷 020 7976 7641
@ pimmune@dial.pipex.com
🖰 www.pia.org.uk

**Princess Mary's Royal Air Force Nursing Service**
✉ c/o Director General
Medical Services (RAF)
HQ PTC RAF Innsworth
Gloucester
GL3 1EZ
☎ 01452 712 612 (Ext 5862)

**Psoriasis Association**
✉ 7 Milton Street
Northampton
NN2 7JG
☎ 01604 711129

## Qualifications and Curriculum Authority (QCA)

✉ 29 Bolton Street
London
W1Y 7PD
☎ 020 7509 5555
🖺 020 7509 6666

## Queen's Nursing Institute

✉ 3 Albermarle Way
London
EC1V 4JB
☎ 020 7490 4227
🖰 www.qni.org.uk

## Registered Nursing Homes Association

✉ Calthorpe House
Hagely Road
Edgbaston
Birmingham
B16 8QY
☎ 0121 454 2511
☎ Freephone: 0800 0740194
🖺 0121 454 0932
🖰 www.rnha.org.uk

## Relate

✉ Herbert Gray College
Little Church Street
Rugby
Warwickshire
CV21 3AP
☎ 01788 573241
🖰 www.relate.org.uk

## Release

✉ The Criminal, Legal and
Drugs Service
388 Old Street
London
EC1V 9CT
☎ 020 7729 9904
🖰 www.release.org.uk

## Research into Ageing

✉ 5–17 St Cross Street
London
EC1N 8UW
☎ 020 7404 6878
🖺 020 7404 6816
@ research@ageing.co.uk
🖰 www.ageing.org

## Royal Association in Aid of Deaf People

✉ Walsingham Road
Colchester
CO2 7BP
☎ 020 8743 6187
🖰 www.info@royaldeaf.org.uk

## Royal College of Anaesthetists

✉ 48–49 Russell Square
London
WC1B 4JY
☎ 020 7813 1888
🖺 020 7636 8280
🖰 www.rcoa.ac.uk

## Royal College of General Practitioners

✉ 14 Princes Gate
Hyde Park
London
SW7 1PU
☎ 020 7581 3232
🖺 020 7589 3145
🖰 http://www.rcgp.org.uk

**Royal College of Midwives**
✉ 15 Mansfield Street
London
W1M 0BE
☎ 020 7312 3535
🖹 020 7312 3561

**Royal College of Nursing of the United Kingdom (RCN)**
✉ 20 Cavendish Square
London
W1M 0AB
☎ 020 7409 3333
🖹 020 7647 3435
🖰 www.rcn.org.uk

**Royal College of Nursing (Northern Ireland)**
✉ 17 Windsor Avenue
Belfast
BT9 6EE
☎ 028 9066 8236
🖹 028 9038 2188
🖰 www.rcn.org.uk

**Royal College of Nursing (Scottish Board)**
✉ 42 South Oswald Road
Edinburgh
EH9 2HH
☎ 0131 662 1010
🖹 0131 662 1032
🖰 www.rcn.org.uk

**Royal College of Nursing (Welsh Board)**
✉ Ty Maeth
King George V Drive
East Cardiff

CF4 4XZ
☎ 02920 751373
🖹 02920 680750

**Royal College of Obstetricians and Gynaecologists**
✉ 27 Sussex Place
Regent's Park
London
NW1 4RG
☎ 020 777 26210
🖹 020 772 30575
🖰 www.rcog.org.uk

**Royal College of Pathologists**
✉ 2 Carlton House Terrace
London
SW1Y 5AF
☎ 020 7451 6700
🖹 020 7451 6701
@ info@rcpath.org

**Royal College of Physicians**
✉ 11 St Andrews Place
London
NW14 LE
☎ 020 7935 1174
🖰 www.rcplondon.ac.uk

**Royal College of Physicians of Edinburgh**
✉ 9 Queen Street
Edinburgh
EH2 1JQ
☎ 0131 225 7324
🖹 0131 220 3939

**Royal College of Psychiatrists**
✉ 17 Belgrave Square
London
SW1X 8PG
☎ 020 7235 2351
🖷 020 7245 1231
🖱 http://www.rcpsych.ac.uk

**Royal College of Radiologists**
✉ 38 Portland Place
London
W1N 3DG
☎ 020 7636 4432
🖱 www.rcr.ac.uk

**Royal College of Speech and Language Therapists**
✉ 2 White Hart Yard
London
SE1 1NX
☎ 020 7378 1200
🖷 020 7403 7254
@ info@rcslt.org
🖱 www.rcslt.org

**Royal College of Surgeons of England**
✉ 35–43 Lincoln's Inn Fields
London
WC2 3PN
☎ 020 7405 3474
🖱 www.rcseng.ac.uk

**Royal Institute of Public Health and Hygiene**
✉ 28 Portland Place
London

W1N 4DE
☎ 020 7580 2731
🖷 020 7580 6157
🖱 www.info@riphh.org.uk

**Royal National Institute for the Blind**
✉ 224 Great Portland Street
London
W1N 6AA
☎ 020 7388 1266
🖱 www.rnib.org.uk

**Royal National Institute for Deaf People**
✉ 19–23 Featherstone Street
London
EC1Y 8SL
☎ 020 7296 8000
🖱 www.rnid.org.uk

**Royal National Pension Fund for Nurses**
✉ Burdett House
15 Buckingham Street
Strand
London
WC2N 6ED
☎ 020 7839 6785
🖱 www.rnpfn.co.uk

**Royal Pharmaceutical Society of Great Britain**
✉ 1 Lambeth High Street
London
SE1 7JN
☎ 020 7735 9141
🖷 020 7735 7629

@ HYPERLINK "mailto: enquiries@rpsgb.org.uk" enquiries@rpsgb.org.uk

### Royal Society of Health
⊠ RSH House
38A St George's Drive
London
SW1V 4BH
① 020 7630 0121
▤ 020 7976 6847
⌇ www.rfph.org

### Royal Society of Medicine (RSM)
⊠ 1 Wimpole Street
London
W1M 8AE
① 020 7290 2900
⌇ www.rsm.ac.uk

### Royal Society for the Prevention of Accidents (ROSPA)
⊠ Edgbaston Park
353 Bristol Road
Birmingham
B5 7ST
① 0121 248 2000
⌇ www.rospa.co.uk

### Sainsbury Centre for Mental Health
⊠ 134–138 Borough High Street
London
SE1 1LB
⌇ www.SainsburyCentre.org.uk

### Samaritans
⊠ 46 Marshall Street
London
W1V 1CR
① 0345 90 90 90
⌇ www.samaritans.org.uk

### Schizophrenia Association of Great Britain
⊠ Bryn Hyfryd
The Crescent
Bangor
Gwynedd
LL57 2AG
① 01248 354048
⌇ www.btinternet.com/~sagb

### Scoliosis Association (UK)
⊠ 2 Ivebury Court
325 Latimer Road
London
W10 6RA
① 020 8964 5343
⌇ www.sauk.org.uk

### Scope
⊠ 6 Market Road
London
N7 9PW
① 020 7619 7100
⌇ www.scope.org.uk

### The Scottish Council on Alcohol
⊠ Second Floor
166 Buchanan Street
Glasgow
G1 2NH
① 0141 333 9677
⌇ Website under construction

## Scottish Council for Single Parents

✉ 13 Gayfield Square
Edinburgh
EH1 3NX
☎ 0131 556 3899
🖰 www.gn.apc.org/opfs

## Scottish Executive

✉ St Andrews House
Regent Road
Edinburgh
EH1 3DG

## Scottish Health Department

✉ St Andrew's House
Regent Road
Edinburgh
EH1 3DG
☎ 0131 556 8400
🖰 www.scotland.gov.uk

## Scottish Health Information Network

🖰 www.shinelib.org.uk

## Scottish Home Department

✉ Saughton House
Broomhouse Drive
Edinburgh
EH11 3XD
☎ 0131 556 8400
🖰 www.scotland.gov.uk

## Shelter (The National Campaign for Homeless People)

✉ 88 Old Street
London
EC1V 9HU

☎ 020 7505 4699
@ info@shelter.org.uk
🖰 www.shelter.org.uk

## Sickle Cell Society

✉ 54 Station Road
Harlesden
London
NW10 4BO
☎ 020 8961 4006
🖰 www.sicklecellsociety.org

## Skin Care Campaign

✉ 163 Eversholt Street
London
NW1 1BU
☎ 020 7388 4097
📄 020 7388 5882
🖰 www.eczema.org

## Smokers Quitline

✉ Victory House
170 Tottenham Court Road
London
W1P 0HA
☎ 020 7487 3000
🖰 www.quit.org.uk

## Society of Chiropodists and Podiatrists

✉ 3 Welbeck Street
London
W1 7HE
☎ 020 7486 3381

## Society and College of Radiographers

✉ 207 Providence Square
Mill Street
London
SE1 2EW

☎ 020 7740 7200
📄 020 7740 7233
🖱 www.sor.org

## Spinal Injuries Association
✉ Newpoint House
76 St James Lane
Muswell Hill
London
N10 3DF
☎ 020 8444 2121
🖱 www.spinal.co.uk

## SPOD (Association to aid the sexual and personal relationships of people with a disability)
✉ 286 Camden Road
London
N7 0BJ
☎ 020 7607 8851
🖱 www.spod.net

## St John Ambulance Association
✉ 1 Grosvenor Crescent
London
SW1X 7EF
☎ 020 7235 5231
🖱 www.sja.org.uk

## Stroke Association
✉ Stroke House
123–127 Whitecross Street
London
EC1Y 8JJ
☎ 020 7490 7999
🖱 www.stroke.org.uk

## Student Nurses' Association
✉ Royal College of Nursing
20 Cavendish Square
London
W1M 0AB
☎ 020 7409 3333
🖱 www.rcn.org.uk

## Tavistock Institute of Human Relations
✉ 30 Tabernacle Street
London
EC2A 4DD
☎ 020 7417 0407
🖱 www.tavistockinstitute.org

## Terrence Higgins Trust
✉ 52–54 Gray's Inn Road
London
WC1X 8JU
☎ 020 7242 1010
🖱 www.tht.org.uk

## Tuberous Sclerosis Association of Great Britain
✉ Little Barnsley Farm
Catshill
Bromsgrove
Worcs.
B61 0NQ
☎ 01527 871898
🖱 www.tuberous-sclerosis.org

## Twins and Multiple Birth Association (TAMBA)
✉ Harnott House
309 Chester Road
Little Sutton

Ellesmere Port
CH66 1QQ
① 0151 348 0020
🖰 www.tamba.org.uk

**UNISON**
🖰 http://www.unison.org.uk

**United Kingdom Central Council for Nursing, Midwifery and Health Visiting**
✉ 23 Portland Place
London
W1B 1PZ
① 020 7637 7181
🖹 020 7436 2924
🖰 www.ukcc.org.uk

**United Kingdom Thalassaemia Society**
✉ 19 The Broadway
Southgate
London
N14 6PH
① 020 8882 0011
🖹 020 8882 8618

**Urostomy Association**
✉ Buckland
Beaumont Park
Danbury
Essex
CM3 4DE
① 01245 224 294
🖰 www.uagbi.org

**Vegan Society**
✉ Donald Watson House

7 Battle Road
St Leonards on Sea
East Sussex
TN37 7AA
① 01424 427393
🖰 www.vegansociety.com

**Victim Support National Association**
✉ Cranmer House
39 Brixton Road
London
SW9 6DZ
① 020 7735 9166
🖰 www.victimsupport.com

**Welsh National Board for Nursing, Midwifery and Health Visiting**
✉ Second Floor
Golate House
101 St Mary Street
Cardiff
CF1 1DX
① 01222 261400
🖹 01222 261499

**Women's Health Concern (WHC)**
✉ 93–99 Upper Richmond Road
London
① 020 8780 3916

**World Health Organisation**
✉ Ave Appia 1211
Geneva 27
Switzerland
① (22) 7912111
🖹 (22) 710746

# Abbreviations

| | |
|---|---|
| AA | Alcoholics Anonymous |
| ACGT | Advisory Committee on Genetic Testing |
| ACHEW | Association of Community Health Councils for England and Wales |
| AFASIC | Association for All Speech Impaired Children |
| AHHRM | Association of Healthcare Human Resource Management |
| AMGP | Association of Managers in General Practice |
| AMRC | Association of Medical Research Charities |
| AMSPAR | Association of Medical Secretaries, Practice Managers, Administrators and Receptionists |
| AP(E)L | Assessment of Prior (Experiential) Learning |
| ASBAH | Association for Spina Bifida and Hydrocephalus |
| ASH | Action for Smoking and Health |
| ASPIRE | Association for Spinal Injury Research, Rehabilitation and Reintegration |
| AVMA | Action for Victims of Medical Accidents |
| | |
| BAC | British Association for Counselling |
| BACUP | British Association for Cancer United Patients |
| BCMA | British Complementary Medicine Association |
| BDA | British Dental Association |
| BGS | British Geriatrics Society |
| BIBIC | British Institute for Brain Injured Children |
| BKPA | British Kidney Patient Association |
| BLISS | Baby Life Support Systems |
| BMA | British Medical Association |
| BODY | British Organ Donor Society |
| BPAS | British Pregnancy Advisory Service |
| BRCS | British Red Cross Society |
| BUPA | British United Provident Association |

| CAF | Contact a Family |
| CAM | Complementary and Alternative Medicine |
| CATS | Credit Accumulation and Transfer Scheme |
| CDNA | Community and District Nursing Association |
| CDP | Community Drug Project |
| CE | Continuing Education |
| CETSW | Council for the Education and Training of Social Workers |
| CHA | Community Hospitals Association |
| CHC | Community Health Councils |
| CHI | Commission for Health Improvement |
| CHIC | Consumer Health Information Centre |
| CNA | Carers National Association |
| COSHH | The Control of Substances Hazardous to Health |
| CPD | Continuing Professional Development |
| CPG | Coronary Prevention Group |
| CPHVA | Community Practitioners and Health Visitors Association |
| CPSM | Council for Professions Supplementary to Medicines |
| | |
| DBCs | Dental Bodies Corporate |
| DBFO | Design, Build, Finance and Operate (contract) |
| DFID | Department for International Development |
| DGs | Directorates General (of the EU) |
| DHSS | Department of Health and Social Services |
| DIAL(UK) | Disablement Information and Advice Line |
| DOH | Department of Health |
| DTI | Department of Trade and Industry |
| | |
| EBP | Evidence based practice |
| EEA | European Economic Area |
| ENB | English National Board for Nursing, Midwifery and Health Visiting |
| EOC | Equal Opportunities Commission |
| EU | European Union |
| | |
| FHSA | Family Health Services Authority |
| FOI | Freedom of Information (Act) |
| | |
| GDC | General Dental Council |
| GIG | Genetic Interest Group |

| | |
|---|---|
| GMC | General Medical Council |
| GOC | General Optical Council |
| GOsC | General Osteopathic Council |
| GSCC | General Social Care Council |
| | |
| HA | Health Authority |
| HAZs | Health Action Zones |
| HCI | Health Coalition Initiative |
| HEA | Health Education Authority |
| HEBS | Health Education Board for Scotland |
| HES | Hospital episode statistics |
| HImPs | Health Improvement Programmes |
| HR | Human resource |
| HRA | Human Rights Act |
| HSC | Health Service Commissioner |
| HSE | Health and Safety Executive |
| HSSB | Health and Social Services Boards |
| HSSE | Health and Social Services Executive (Northern Ireland) |
| | |
| ICAN | Invalid Children's Aid Nationwide |
| ICN | International Council of Nurses |
| ICRF | Imperial Cancer Research Fund |
| IEHO | Institute of Environmental Health Officers |
| IHA | Independent Healthcare Association |
| IHSM | Institute of Health Service Managers |
| IM&T | Information Management and Technology (systems) |
| | |
| JIPs | Joint investment plans |
| | |
| LMCA | The Long-term Medical Conditions Alliance |
| | |
| MCA | Medicines Control Agency |
| MCNs | Managed Clinical Networks |
| MDU | Medical Defence Union |
| MEPs | Members of the European Parliament |
| MSF | Manufacturing Science and Finance |
| | |
| NAHAT | National Association of Health Authorities and Trusts |
| NBA | National Blood Authority |

| NBNI | National Board for Nursing, Midwifery and Health Visiting for Northern Ireland |
| NBS | National Board for Nursing, Midwifery and Health Visiting for Scotland |
| NCSC | National Care Standards Commission |
| NCT | National Childbirth Trust |
| NeLH | National electronic Library for Health |
| NHS | National Health Service |
| NHSE | National Health Service Executive |
| NHS IM&T | National Health Service Information Management & Technology |
| NICE | National Institute of Clinical Excellence |
| NIF | National Information Forum |
| NMC | Nursing and Midwifery Council |
| NNA | Neonatal Nurses Association |
| NPAT | National Patients' Access Team |
| NRPB | National Radiographic Protection Board |
| NSC | National Screening Committee |
| NSF | National Schizophrenia Fellowship |
| NSFs | National service frameworks |
| NSPCC | National Society for the Prevention of Cruelty to Children |
| NVQ | National Vocational Qualification |
| | |
| PAF | Performance Assessment Framework |
| PALS | Patient Advocacy and Liaison Service |
| PAMS | Professions allied to medicine |
| PCG | Primary Care Group |
| PCT | Primary Care Trust |
| PFI | Private Finance Initiative |
| PIA | Primary Immunodeficiency Association |
| PIF | Patient Information Forum |
| PMS | Personal Medical Services |
| PREP | Post-Registration Education and Practice |
| | |
| QCA | Qualifications and Curriculum Authority |
| QNI | Queen's Nursing Institute |
| | |
| RCN | Royal College of Nursing |
| RIPHH | Royal Institute of Public Health and Hygiene |

| | |
|---|---|
| RNHA | Registered Nursing Home Association |
| ROSPA | Royal Society for the Prevention of Accidents |
| RSH | Royal Society of Health |
| RSM | Royal Society of Medicine |
| RTC | Regional Transfusion Centre |
| | |
| SaFFs | Service and Financial Frameworks |
| SCOTVEC | Scottish Vocational and Education Council |
| SEB | Scottish Examining Board |
| SHINE | Scottish Health Information Network |
| SI | Statutory Instrument |
| SIGN | Scottish Intercollegiate Guidelines Network |
| SPOD | Association to aid the sexual and personal relationships of people with a disability |
| SPV | Special purpose vehicle |
| SQA | Scottish Qualifications Authority |
| STUC | Scottish Trades Union Congress |
| SVQ | Scottish Vocational Qualification |
| | |
| TAMBA | Twins and Multiple Birth Association |
| TUC | Trades Union Congress |
| TUPE | Transfer of Undertakings (Protection of Employment) |
| | |
| UKCC | United Kingdom Council for Nursing, Midwifery and Health Visiting |
| | |
| WHC | Women's Health Concern |
| WHCSA | Welsh Health Common Services Agency |
| WHO | World Health Organisation |
| WNB | Welsh National Board for Nursing, Midwifery and Health Visiting |

# Health related reports, inquiries, Green Papers and White Papers: short and official titles

This is an alphabetical list of the short, 'popular' titles by which official health-related reports, Green Papers, White Papers and Acts of Parliament are often known. These short titles are often derived from the name of the person who chaired the group or committee who produced the report. Each entry provides the item's full title and further bibliographic details. If items share a popular title, entries are arranged in chronological order.

**Acheson Report**
*Report of the independent inquiry into inequalities in health*
London: Stationery Office, 1998 ISBN: 0113221738

**Acheson Report**
*Public health in England: the report of the committee of inquiry into the future development of the public health function* (Cm 289)
London: HMSO, 1988

**Allitt Inquiry**
*Independent inquiry relating to deaths and injuries on the children's ward at Grantham and Kesteven General Hospital*
London: HMSO, 1994
This is also known as the Clothier Report

**Ashton Report**
*Review of the Cardiac Unit at the Royal Liverpool Children's Hospital NHS Trust Alder Hey*
NHS Executive North West, 2000

**Banks Review**
Coopers and Lybrand
*Review of the wider Department of Health*
London: DOH, 1994

**Barlow Report**
*Report of the advisory group on osteoporosis*
London: DOH, 1994

**Bevan Report**
*Staffing and utilisation of operating theatres*
London: HMSO, 1989

**Beveridge Report**
*Social insurance and allied services: report* (Cmd 6404)
London: HMSO, 1942  ISBN: 0108502767

**Black Report**
*Inequalities in health: report of a research working group*
London: DHSS, 1980
Revised editions have since been published by Penguin in 1982,
1988 and 1992

**Blom Cooper Report**
*Report of the committee of inquiry into complaints about Ashworth
Hospital*
London: HMSO, 1992
Vol 1 (Cm 2028I)  ISBN: 010202822
Vol 2: Case studies (Cm 2028II)  ISBN: 010202830

**Bonham-Carter Report**
*Functions of the District General Hospitals*
London: HMSO, 1969

**Boyd Report**
Department of Health
*Confidential inquiry into homicides and suicides by mentally ill people*
London: HMSO, 1994

**Bradbeer Report**
*Internal administration of hospitals*
London: HMSO, 1954

**Briggs Report**
*Report of the committee on nursing* (Cmnd 5115)
London: HMSO, 1972

**Butler Report**
*Report of the committee on mentally abnormal offenders* (Cmnd 6244)
London: HMSO, 1975

**Butterworth Report**
Mental Health Nursing Review Team
*Working in partnership: a collaborative approach to care*
London: HMSO, 1994

**Caldicott Committee Report**
*Report on the review of patient-identifiable information*
London: NHS Executive, 1997

**Calman Report**
*Junior doctors: the new deal*
London: HMSO, 1991

**Calman Report**
*Hospital doctors' training for the future: the report of the working group on specialist medical training*
London: DOH, 1993.

**Calman-Hine Report**
Expert Advisory Group on Cancer to the Chief Medical Officers of England and Wales
*A policy framework for commissioning cancer services*
DOH and Welsh Office, 1995

**Canterbury Report**
Health Education Council. Steering Committee
*Coronary heart disease prevention: plans for action: a report based on an interdisciplinary workshop conference held at Canterbury on 28–30 September 1983*
London: Pitman, 1984  ISBN: 0272797989

**Cave Report**
*Voluntary hospitals and their services: interim report* (Cmd 1206)
London: Ministry of Health, 1921

### Cave Report
*Voluntary hospitals and their services: final report* (Cmd 1335)
London: Ministry of Health, 1921

### Ceri Davies Report
*Under-used and surplus property in the National Health Service: report of an enquiry into ways of identifying surplus land and property in the National Health Service*
London: DHSS, 1983 ISBN: 0113208278

### Clothier Report
Department of Health and Social Security
*Report of the committee appointed to inquire into the circumstances, including the production, which led to the use of contaminated infusion fluids in the Devonport section of Plymouth General Hospital*
London: HMSO, 1972 ISBN: 0101503504

### Clothier Report
*Independent inquiry relating to deaths and injuries on the children's ward at Grantham and Kesteven General Hospital*
London: HMSO, 1994
This is the report of the Allitt Inquiry

### Cogwheel Reports
*First report of the joint working party on the organisation of medical work in hospitals*
London: HMSO, 1967
*Second report of the joint working party on the organisation of medical work in hospitals*
*Third report of the joint working party on the organisation of medical work in hospitals*
London: HMSO, 1974

### Collins Report
Collins, J
*When the eagles fly: a report on resettlement of people with learning difficulties from long-stay institutions*
London: Values into Action, 1992

### Community Care Act
*National Health Service and Community Care Act 1990*
London: HMSO, 1990

**Court Report**
*Fit for the future: report of the committee on child health services*
(Cmnd 6684)
London: HMSO, 1976

**Cranbrook Report**
*Report of the maternity services committee*
London: HMSO, 1959

**Crown Report**
*Report of the advisory group on nurse prescribing*
London: DOH, 1989

**Cullen Report**
Chief Nursing Officers of the UK
*Caring for people: mental handicap nursing*
(PL/CNO (91) 5)
London: DOH, 1991

**Culyer Report**
Culyer, A
*Supporting research and development in the NHS: a report to the Minister of Health*
London: HMSO, 1994  ISBN: 0113218311

**Cumberlege Report**
*Neighbourhood nursing: a focus for care*
London: HMSO, 1986

**Cumberlege Report**
DOH. Expert Maternity Group
*Changing childbirth*
London: HMSO, 1993 (2 vols)  ISBN: 0113216238

**Curtis Report**
*Report of the care of children committee* (Cmd 6922)
London: HMSO, 1946

**Davies Report**
*Report of the committee on hospital complaints procedure*
London: HMSO, 1973  ISBN: 0113205317

**Dawson Report**
Consultative Council on Medical and Allied Services
*Interim report on the future provision of medical and allied services*
(Cmd 693)
London: HMSO, 1920

**Dowie Reports**
Dowie, R
*Patterns of hospital medical staffing*
London: HMSO, 1991
A series of nine reports:

1. Overview
2. Anaesthetics
3. General Medicine
4. General Psychiatry
5. General Surgery
6. Obstetrics and Gynaecology
7. Ophthalmology
8. Paediatrics
9. Trauma and Orthopaedic Surgery

**Duthie Report**
Joint Subcommittee of the Standing Medical, Nursing and Midwifery, and Pharmaceutical Advisory Committees
*Guidelines for the safe and secure handling of medicines: a report to the Secretary of State for Social Services*
London: DOH, 1988

**Fallon Report**
*Report of the committee of inquiry into the Personality Disorder Unit, Ashworth Special Hospital* (Cm 4194-II)
London: Stationery Office, 1999  ISBN: 0101419430
*Volume II: Expert evidence on personality disorder* (Cm 4195)
London: Stationery Office, 1999  ISBN: 01041952

**Farquharson-Lang Report**
*Administrative practice of hospital boards in Scotland*
Edinburgh: HMSO, 1966

**First Green Paper**
*Administrative structure of the medical and related services in England and Wales*
London: HMSO, 1968

**Firth Report**
*Public support for residential care: report of a joint central and local government working party*
London: DHSS, 1987

**Forrest Report**
*Breast cancer screening: report to the health ministers of England, Wales, Scotland and Northern Ireland*
London: HMSO, 1986  ISBN: 011321071X

**Glancy Report**
*Revised report of the working party on security in NHS psychiatric hospitals*
London: HMSO, 1974

**Goodenough Report**
*Report of the inter-departmental committee on medical schools*
London: Ministry of Health, 1944  ISBN: 0946539014

**Green Paper**
*National Health Service: the future structure of the National Health Service in England*
London: HMSO, 1970  ISBN: 113209959

**Green Paper**
*Primary health care: an agenda for discussion* (Cmnd 9771)
London: HMSO, 1986

**Green Paper**
*Health of the nation: a consultative document for health in England* (Cm 1523)
London: HMSO, 1991  ISBN: 0101152329

**Griffiths Report**
*National Health Service management inquiry report*
London: DHSS, 1984  ISBN: 0946539014

### Griffiths Report
*Community care: agenda for action*
London: HMSO, 1988  ISBN: 0113211309

### Guillebaud Report
*Cost of the National Health Service: report of the committee of enquiry*
London: HMSO, 1956

### Hall Reports
*Report of the joint working party on child health surveillance: health for all children*
Hall, DMB (ed)
1st edn 1989
2nd edn 1991
3rd edn OUP 1996

### Halsbury Report
*Report of the committee of inquiry into the pay and related conditions of service of nurses and midwives*
London: HMSO, 1974

### Halsbury Report
*Report of the committee of inquiry into the pay and related conditions of service of the professions supplementary to medicine and speech therapists*
London: HMSO, 1975

### Harding Report
*The primary health care team: report of a joint working group of the Standing Medical Advisory Committee and the Standing Nursing and Midwifery Advisory Committee*
London: DHSS, 1981

### Harvard Davies Report
*The organisation of group practice: report of a sub-committee of the Standing Medical Advisory Committee*
London: HMSO, 1971

### Heathrow Debate
*The challenges for nursing and midwifery in the 21st century: a report of the Heathrow debate between chief nursing officers of England, Wales, Scotland and Northern Ireland* (held in May 1993)
London: HMSO, 1994

## Hill Report
*Hospital treatment of acute poisoning: report of the joint sub-committee of the Standing Medical Advisory Committee. Central and Scottish Health Councils.*
London: DHSS, 1968

## Hinchliffe Report
*Final report of the committee on the cost of prescribing*
London: HMSO, 1959

## Hunt Report
*Report of the committee on hospital supplies organisation*
Circulated to hospital authorities under cover of HM (66) 69

## Hunter Report
*Report of the working party on medical administrators*
London: HMSO, 1972

## Ingall Report
*Training of district nurses. Report of the Advisory Committee*
London: Ministry of Health, 1958

## Jay Report
*Report of the committee of enquiry into mental handicap nursing and care* (Cmnd 7468)
London: HMSO, 1979 (2 vols)

## Judge Report
Commission on Nursing Education
*The education of nurses: a new dispensation*
London: Royal College of Nursing, 1985

## Körner Report
*First report of the steering group on health services information*
London: HMSO, 1982

## Lewin Report
*Organisation and staffing of operating departments*
London: HMSO, 1970

**Limerick Report**
*Expert group to investigate cot death theories: toxic gas hypothesis final report*
London: DOH, 1998  ISBN: 1858398746

**Lung Report**
British Lung Foundation
*Lung disease: a shadow over the nation's health*
London: British Lung Foundation, 1996  ISBN: 0952747200

**Lycett Green Report**
*Report of the committee of enquiry into the recruitment, training and promotion of administrative and clerical staff in the hospital service*
London: HMSO, 1963

**Mansell Report**
*Services for people with learning disabilities and challenging behaviour or mental health needs: report of a project group*
London: HMSO, 1993  ISBN: 011321569

**Mant Report**
*Research and development in primary care: national working group report*
Leeds: NHSE, 1998

**McCarthy Report**
*Making Whitley work*
Edinburgh: DHSS, 1976

**McColl Report**
*Review of artificial limb and appliance centre services*
Edinburgh: HMSO, 1986

**Merrison Report**
*Report of the committee of inquiry into the regulation of the medical profession* (Cmnd 6018)
London: HMSO, 1975

**Merrison Report**
*Royal Commission on the National Health Service* (Cmnd 7615)
London: HMSO, 1979

**Monks Report**
*Report of the working group to examine workloads in genito-urinary medicine clinics*
London: DOH, 1988

**Montgomery Report**
*Maternity services in Scotland*
Edinburgh: HMSO, 1959

**Nodder Report**
*Organisational and management problems of mental illness hospitals: report of a working group*
London: DHSS, 1980

**Noel Hall Report**
*Grading structure of the administrative and clerical staff in the hospital service*
London: HMSO, 1957

**Noel Hall Report**
*Report of the working party on the hospital pharmaceutical service*
London: HMSO, 1978

**Omega File**
Adam Smith Institute
*Health and social services policy*
London: Adam Smith Institute, 1984  ISBN: 0906517575

**Peach Report**
UKCC Commission for Nursing and Midwifery and Education
*Fitness for practice*
London: UKCC, 1999

**Peel Report**
Standing Maternity and Midwifery Advisory Committee
*Domiciliary midwifery and maternity bed needs: report of a sub-committee*
London: HMSO, 1970  ISBN: 0113202563

**Peel Report**
*The use of fetuses and fetal material for research*
London: HMSO, 1972

### Pennington Report
Pennington Group
*Report on the circumstances leading to the 1996 outbreak of infection with E. Coli 0157 in central Scotland, the implications for food safety and the lessons to be learned*
London: Stationery Office, 1997  ISBN: 0114958513

### Pilkington Report
*Royal Commission on doctors' and dentists' remuneration. Report* (Cmnd 939)
London: HMSO, 1960

### Platt Report
*The welfare of children in hospital: report of a committee of the Central Health Services Council*
London: HMSO, 1959

### Polkinghorne Report
*Review of the guidance on the research use of fetuses and fetal material*
London: HMSO, 1972

### Powell Report
Central Health Services Council. Ministry of Health
*Report of the sub-committee appointed to answer the pattern of the inpatients' day* (Cmd 7402)
London: HMSO, 1946

### RAWP Report
Resource Allocation Working Party
*Sharing resources for health in England*
London: HMSO, 1976

### Red Book
DOH and Welsh Office
*Statement of fees and allowances payable to general medical practitioners in England and Wales from 1 April 1990*
London: HMSO, 1992

### Reed Report
*Review of mental health and social services for mentally disordered offenders and others requiring similar services: vol 1: final summary report* (Cm 2088)
London: HMSO, 1992  ISBN: 0101208820

**Reed Report**
*Review of mental health and social services for mentally disordered offenders and others requiring similar services: vol 2: service needs*
London: HMSO, 1993 ISBN: 0113215517

**Reed Report**
*Review of mental health and social services for mentally disordered offenders and others requiring similar services: vol 3: finance, staffing and training*
London: HMSO, 1993 ISBN: 0113215525

**Reed Report**
*Review of mental health and social services for mentally disordered offenders and others requiring similar services: vol 4: the academic and research base*
London: HMSO, 1993 ISBN: 0113215533

**Reed Report**
*Review of mental health and social services for mentally disordered offenders and others requiring similar services: vol 5: special issues and differing needs*
London: HMSO, 1993 ISBN: 0113215541

**Reed Report**
*High security and related psychiatric provision*
London: HMSO, 1994

**Reed Report**
*Services for people with psychopathic disorder*
London: HMSO, 1994

**Richards Report**
*Clinical academic careers: report of an independent task force chaired by Sir Rex Richards*
London: Committee of Vice-Chancellors and Principals of the Universities of the UK, 1997

**Ritchie Report**
*Report of the inquiry into the care and treatment of Christopher Clunis*
London: HMSO, 1994 ISBN: 0117017981

**Ritchie Report**
*Report of the inquiry into quality and practice within the National Health Service arising from the actions of Rodney Ledward*
London: DOH, 2000

**Rothschild Report**
*The organisation and management of government research and development* (Cmnd 4814)
London: HMSO, 1971

**Rothschild Report**
*A framework for government research and development* (Cmnd 5046)
London: HMSO, 1972

**Rubery Report**
*Report of the Chief Medical Officer's expert group on the sleeping position of infants and cot deaths*
London: HMSO, 1993  ISBN: 011321605x

**Sainsbury Report**
*Report of the committee of inquiry into the relationship of the pharmaceutical industry with the National Health Service* (Cmnd 3410)
London: HMSO, 1967

**Salmon Report**
*Report of the committee on senior nursing staff structure*
London: HMSO, 1966

**SCHARR Report**
Reed, S
*Catching the tide: new voyages in nursing*
Sheffield: University of Sheffield, Sheffield Centre for Health and Related Research, 1995
This became known as the SCHARR Report after it was referred to as such in Executive Letter 95/98, September 1995. SCHARR have since produced many reports.

**Schofield Report**
University of Manchester. Health Services Management Unit. Project Steering Group

*The future healthcare workforce: the steering group report*
Manchester: HSMU, 1996  ISBN: 0946250073

**Scottish Green Paper**
*Administrative reorganisation of the Scottish health services*
London: HMSO, 1968

**Second Green Paper**
*National Health Service: the future structure of the National Health Service in England*
London: HMSO, 1970

**Seebohm Report**
*Report by the committee on local authority and allied social services*
London: HMSO, 1968

**Sheldon Report**
*Report of the expert group on special care babies*
London: HMSO, 1971

**Shields Report**
Scottish Office. Department of Health. Working Group on the Roles and Responsibilities of Health Boards
*Commissioning better health: report of the short life working group on the roles and responsibilities of health boards*
Edinburgh: Scottish Office, 1996

**Short Report**
*Second report from the Social Services Committee. Perinatal and neonatal mortality* (Session 1979/80, HC 663)
London: HMSO, 1980  ISBN: 0102976805

**Short Report**
*Third report from the Social Services Committee. Perinatal and neonatal mortality, follow up* (Session 1983/84, HC 308)
London: HMSO, 1984  ISBN: 0102308845

**Spens Report**
*Report of the inter-departmental committee on the remuneration of general practitioners* (Cmd 6810)
London: HMSO, 1946

**Spens Report**
*Report of the inter-departmental committee on the remuneration of general dental practitioners* (Cmd 7402)
London: HMSO, 1948

**Tilt Report**
*Report of the review of security at the high security hospitals*
London: DOH, 2000

**Todd Report**
*Report of the Royal Commission on medical education* (Cmnd 3569)
London: HMSO, 1968

**Tomlinson Report**
*Report of the inquiry into London's health service, medical education and research*
London: HMSO, 1992  ISBN: 0113215487

**Tunbridge Report**
*The care of the health of hospital staff. Report of the Joint Committee of the Central and Scottish Health Services Councils*
London: HMSO, 1968

**Turnberg Report**
*Health services in London: a strategic review*
London: DOH, 1998

**Turner Report**
*Sudden infant death syndrome: report of the expert working group enquiring into the hypothesis that toxic gases evolved from chemicals in cot mattress covers and cot mattresses are a cause of SIDS*
London: HMSO, 1991  ISBN: 0952747200

**Utting Report**
*Children in the public care: a review of residential care*
London: HMSO, 1991  ISBN: 0113214553

**Warnock Report**
*Report of the committee of inquiry into human fertilisation and embryology* (Cmnd 9314)
London: HMSO, 1984  ISBN: 0101931409

**Welsh Green Paper**
*Reorganisation of the health service in Wales*

**White Paper**
*NHS reorganisation England* (Cmnd 5055)
London: HMSO, 1972

**White Paper**
*Prevention and Health* (Cmnd 7047)
London: HMSO, 1977

**White Paper**
*Growing older* (Cmnd 8173)
London: HMSO, 1981

**White Paper**
*Promoting better health: the Government's programme for improving primary health care* (Cm 249)
London: HMSO, 1987  ISBN: 0101024924

**White Paper**
*Caring for people: community care in the next decade and beyond* (Cm 849)
London: HMSO, 1989

**White Paper**
DOH
*Working for patients* (Cm 555)
London: HMSO, 1989  ISBN: 0101055528

**White Paper**
*Primary care: delivering the future* (Cm 3512)
London: HMSO, 1991  ISBN: 0101351224

**White Paper**
*Health of the nation: a strategy for health in England* (Cm 1986)
London: HMSO, 1992  ISBN: 0101198620

**White Paper**
*Choice and opportunity – primary care: the future* (Cm 3390)
London: HMSO, 1996  ISBN: 010133902x

**Winterton Report**
House of Commons Health Select Committee
*Second report on the maternity services*
*Vol 1: Report together with appendices and the proceedings of the Committee* ISBN: 0102830924
*Vol 2: Minutes of evidence* ISBN: 0102838925
*Vol 3: Appendices to the minutes of evidence* ISBN: 0102897921
London: HMSO, 1992

**Woodbine Parish Report**
*Hospital building maintenance: report of the committee, 1968–1970*
London: HMSO, 1970 ISBN: 0113209924

**Zuckerman Report**
*Hospital scientific and technical services*
London: HMSO, 1968

# Degrees, diplomas and organisations: abbreviations in healthcare

| | |
|---|---|
| AA | Alcoholics Anonymous |
| ABPN | Association of British Paediatric Nurses |
| AIMSW | Association of the Institute of Medical Social Workers |
| AOC | Aromatherapy Organisations Council |
| APEX | Association of Professional and Executive Staffs |
| ASH | Action on Smoking and Health |
| | |
| BA | Bachelor of Arts |
| BACUP | British Association of Cancer United Patients |
| BAON | British Association of Orthopaedic Nurses |
| BDA | British Dental Association |
| BDSc | Bachelor of Dental Science |
| BEd | Bachelor of Education |
| BITA | British Intravenous Therapy Association |
| BMAS | British Medical Acupuncture Society |
| BN | Bachelor of Nursing |
| BPOG | British Psychosocial Oncology Group |
| BRA | British Reflexology Association |
| BRCS | British Red Cross Society |
| BSc (Soc Sci-Nurs) | Bachelor of Science (Nursing) |
| BSMDH | British Society of Medical and Dental Hypnosis |
| | |
| CATS | Credit Accumulation Transfer Scheme |
| CCETSW | Central Council for Educational Training in Social Work |
| CCHE | Central Council for Health Education |

| CMT | Clinical Midwife Teacher |
| CNF | Commonwealth Nurses Federation |
| CNN | Certificated Nursery Nurse |
| COSHH | Control of Substances Hazardous to Health |
| CSP | Chartered Society of Physiotherapists |
| | |
| DCH | Diploma in Child Health |
| DDA | Dangerous Drugs Act |
| DipAr | Diploma in Aromatherapy |
| DipEd | Diploma in Education |
| DipHyp | Diploma in Hypnotherapy |
| DipMedAc | Diploma in Medical Acupuncture |
| Dip NE | Diploma in Nursing Education |
| Dip NEd | Diploma in Nursing Education |
| DipPhyto | Diploma in Phytotherapy |
| DN | Diploma in Nursing |
| DNA | District Nursing Association |
| DOH | Department of Health |
| DPH | Diploma in Public Health |
| DPhil | Doctor of Philosophy |
| DPM | Diploma in Psychological Medicine |
| DSc | Doctor of Science |
| DTM&H | Diploma in Tropical Medicine and Hygiene |
| | |
| EN | Enrolled Nurse |
| ENB | English National Board for Nursing, Midwifery and Health Visiting |
| | |
| FCSP | Fellow of the Chartered Society of Physiotherapists |
| FETC | Further Education Teaching Certificate |
| FNIF | Florence Nightingale International Foundation |
| FNIMH | Fellow of National Institute of Medical Herbalists |
| fpa | Family Planning Association |
| FRCN | Fellow of the Royal College of Nursing |
| FRS | Fellow of the Royal Society |
| FRSH | Fellow of the Royal Society of Health |

| | |
|---|---|
| GMC | General Medical Council |
| GNVQ | General National Vocational Qualification |
| HAS | Hospital Savings Association |
| HEA | Health Education Authority |
| HFEA | Human Fertilisation and Embryology Authority |
| HV | Health Visitor |
| ICN | International Council of Nurses |
| ICNA | Infection Control Nurses Association |
| ICW | International Council of Women |
| IFA | International Federation of Aromatherapists |
| IHF | International Hospital Federation |
| INR | Index of Nursing Research |
| LFHom | Licensed Associate of the Faculty of Homeopathy |
| MA | Master of Arts |
| MAACP | Member of Acupuncture Association of Chartered Physiotherapists |
| MAO | Master of the Art of Obstetrics |
| MAOT | Member of the Association of Occupational Therapists |
| MBA | Master of Business Administration |
| MBAC | Member of British Acupuncture Council |
| MBIM | Member of the British Institute of Management |
| MCSP | Member of the Chartered Society of Physiotherapists |
| MFHom | Member of the Faculty of Homeopathy |
| MIND | National Association for Mental Health |
| MMAA | Member of Modern Acupuncture Association |
| MPhil | Master of Philosophy |
| MRC | Medical Research Council |
| MRSH | Member of the Royal Society of Health |
| MRSHom | Member of the Royal Society of Homeopaths |
| MRSS | Member of Register of Shiatsu Society |
| MSc | Master of Science |
| MSF | Manufacturing Science and Finance |

| | |
|---|---|
| MSRG | Member of the Society of Remedial Gymnasts |
| MSR (R) | Member of the Society of Radiographers (Radiotherapy) |
| MTD | Midwife Teachers' Diploma |
| NAMCW | National Association for Maternal and Child Welfare |
| NAMH | National Association for Mental Health |
| NATN | National Association for Theatre Nurses |
| NAWCH | National Association for the Welfare of Children in Hospital |
| NHS | National Health Service |
| NIB | Northern Ireland Board for Nursing, Midwifery and Health Visiting |
| NIMH | National Institute of Medical Herbalists |
| NNA | Neonatal Nurses Association |
| NNEB | National Nursery Education Board |
| NUMINE | Network of Users of Microcomputers in Nurse Education |
| NUS | National Union of Students |
| NVQ | National Vocational Qualification |
| OHNC | Occupational Health Nursing Certificate |
| ONC | Orthopaedic Nurses' Certificate |
| OND | Ophthalmic Nursing Diploma |
| OT | Occupational Therapist |
| PhD | Doctor of Philosophy |
| PMRAFNS | Princess Mary's Royal Air Force Nursing Service |
| PNA | Psychiatric Nurses' Association |
| ProfDipAr | Professional Diploma in Aromatherapy |
| QARANC | Queen Alexandra's Royal Army Nursing Corps |
| QARNNS | Queen Alexandra's Royal Naval Nursing Service |
| QIDN | Queen's Institute of District Nursing |
| QNI | Queen's Nursing Institute |

| | |
|---|---|
| RCM | Royal College of Midwives |
| RCN | Royal College of Nursing |
| RGN | Registered General Nurse |
| RHV | Regional Health Visitor |
| RM | Registered Midwife |
| RMN | Registered Mental Nurse |
| RN | Registered Nurse |
| RNMH | Registered Nurse for the Mentally Handicapped |
| RNT | Registered Nurse Tutor |
| RSCN | Registered Sick Children's Nurse |
| | |
| StAAA | St Andrew's Ambulance Association |
| StJAA | St John Ambulance Association |
| StJAB | St John Ambulance Brigade |
| SCM | State Certified Midwife |
| SHHD | Scottish Home and Health Department |
| SNB | Scottish National Board for Nursing, Midwifery and Health Visiting |
| SNNEB | Scottish National Nursing Examination Board |
| SRN | State Registered Nurse |
| SSStJ | Serving Sister of the Order of St John of Jerusalem |
| ST | Speech Therapist |
| | |
| UKCC | United Kingdom Central Council for Nursing, Midwifery and Health Visiting |
| VSO | Voluntary Service Overseas |
| | |
| WFH | World Federation of Hypnotherapists |
| WHO | World Health Organisation |
| WNB | Welsh National Board for Nursing, Midwifery and Health Visiting |
| WRVS | Women's Royal Voluntary Service |

# Healthcare on the Internet

For the healthcare professional, the Internet provides a veritable treasure chest of information, but mixed in with the nuggets of gold is a vast amount of irrelevant or useless data. Many hours can be wasted searching for the precise information you require, so the trick is to learn to navigate the Net without too much frustration.

The various types of information accessible via the Web include:

- Information about professional organisations, academic institutions and hospitals, e.g. the Royal College of Nursing.
- Full text or abstracts of many published articles – available through Medline. In addition many journals are now accessible online, either free of charge or on a subscription basis.
- Information about disease states, e.g. AIDS Insite (http://hivinsite.ucsf.edu/).
- Information about drugs.
- Support groups for parents, e.g. websites for parents of premature infants (http://www2.medsch.wisc.edu/childrenshosp/parents_of_preemies/toc.html).
- Details of conferences.

In fact, information on almost any topic is probably now available electronically if you know where to find it.

If you do not know the URL or 'address' of the Web page you want to access, then you need to use one of the search engines such as Yahoo or AltaVista, which should be easily accessible via your browser (e.g. Netscape Navigator or Microsoft Internet Explorer).

When you type in a keyword for the site you want to access, the search engine will bring up a list of all the sites on the Web containing that particular keyword.

Once you have found a site which interests you make sure you bookmark it so that you can find it again. Many sites include links to related websites and these are a good source of high quality information.

To help you find your way around the World Wide Web, listed below are some nursing sites which you may find useful, but do bear in mind that sites are constantly being added and deleted so you will need to do your own research.

**Medisearch**

To focus on the large amount of useful health information there is on the Internet, the UK search engine Mirago has launched a special service called Medisearch (www.medisearch.co.uk), which offers search services for 'authoritative' medical information.

The documents categorised by the Mirago robots as containing medical resources have been compiled in conjunction with UK health professionals, who have classified sites considered to be repositories of 'authoritative' medical information. These resources include UK and international professional, research, administrative, charitable, support and commercial sites in both the public and private sectors. The Medisearch index encompasses hundreds of thousands of pages on health-related topics with the index completely refreshed every 2–3 weeks.

Apart from a free searchable service for health professionals and patients, Medisearch offers news and topic-oriented Web guides linking to thousands of useful health-related sites.

**American Association of Colleges of Nursing (AACN) (http://www.aacn.nche.edu/index.html)**

The site is the Web homepage of the AACN, the national voice of America's university and higher degree nursing education programmes. For members only there is an interactive issues forum.

**Community Practitioners' and Health Visitors' Association (CPHVA) (http://www.msfcphva.org)**

The CPHVA is the UK professional body that represents registered nurses and health visitors who work in primary or community health settings.

**English National Board for Nursing, Midwifery and Health Visiting (ENB) Link Home Page (http://www.enb.org.uk)**

This site aims to disseminate Board information to nurses, midwives and health visitors in England and includes details of current circulars, courses and contact information. There are links to Research Digest listing, the commissioned research and the ENB Health Care Database of nursing literature abstracts.

### Government and official health documents
### (http://www.herts.ac.uk/lis/subjects/health/offdoc.htm)

This site, produced by the Learning and Information Services Department of the University of Hertfordshire, give details of government and official health-related documents available in full text on the Web since 1997. They include:

- Department of Health publications
- Audit Commission reports
- Health Select Committee reports
- Health Service Ombudsman reports
- National Audit Office publications
- World Health Organization publications.

### Health Development Agency
### (http://hda-online.org.uk)

The site is the Web homepage of the Health Development Agency (HDA) which was set up in 2000 to replace the Health Education Authority. It maintains the following websites:

- Arts and community participation for health
- Food and low income database
- HAZnet
- Health at Work in the NHS
- Health Development Agency
- HealthProm*is*
- LifeBytes
- Mind, Body and Soul
- National HIV Prevention Information Service
- Our Healthier Nation
- Quick
- Wired for Health
- Young People's Health Network.

### Index Medicus
### (http://www.medscape.com/Home/Search/Index Medicus)

A full list of journal abbreviations used for Index Medicus.

### Medscape
### (http:www.medscape.com)

Medscape permits free access to full text of a selection of peer-reviewed journals as well as the latest news in different specialties. Registration is required. It also gives free access to Medline.

### Medscape – Drug Information
### (http://www.medscape.com/misc/formdrugs.html)

This site gives information on more than 200 000 prescription and over-the-counter drugs including indications, interactions and precautions. The site also enables you to find drugs to treat a disease and includes an online medical dictionary.

### Mining Co Guide to Nursing
### (http://nursing.miningco.com)

This site is a useful resource for nurses offering Net links, features, bulletin boards, chat and a free newsletter. There are also further links to an evolving index of Net resources on nursing divided by specialty.

### National Board for Nursing, Midwifery and Health Visiting for Northern Ireland
### (http://www.n-i.nhs.uk/NBNI/index.htm)

The site provides advice and information on training for nurses, midwives and health visitors in Northern Ireland.

### National Board for Nursing, Midwifery and Health Visiting for Scotland
### (http://www.nbs.org.uk)

The Board is responsible for standards of education and training for nurses, midwives and health visitors in Scotland. Provides career information for these professions.

### National League for Nursing (NLN)
### (http://www.nln.org/)

The NLN aims to promote quality nursing education in the USA. Information is provided on membership, accreditation programmes, career and education opportunities, as well as news and events.

**Nurses on the Web**
**(http://www.cp-tel.net/pamnorth/webnurse.htm)**
This is a nursing site designed to bring both students and professional nurses together to offer support, communication and assistance. The pages are frequently updated and include information on nursing journals, nursing practice and further nursing links.

**Nursing Around the World**
**(http://www.nurse-dk.com/)**
This is a free access site offering online chat, the Nursing Forums, the Nursing Connection and reviews. A world nurse list allows members to read or debate global nursing issues with nurses internationally.

**Nursing Connection**
**(http:www.nursecon.htm)**
This site provides free listing services for nurses around the world. Each listing includes an email link as well as a description of the individual's interests, location and specialty.

**Nursing (Medicine)**
**(http://www.galaxy.com/cgi-bin/dirlist?node=25254)**
This is a directory of nursing resources with links to nursing research, theory and specialties. There are further links to USA organisations and nursing directories.

**PubMed**
**(http://www.ncbi.nlminih.gov/PubMed)**
This is the National Library of Medicine's free search service with access to 9 million citations in Medline with links to participating online journals.

**Raven's Child – Nursing Links**
**(http://home.att.net/~ravenschild/)**
This site has homepage linking to sites on community health nursing, ICU nursing and trauma. This site is designed as a resource for students, nurses and other medical personnel.

**Royal College of Nursing Conference and Exhibition Unit**
**(http://nursing-standard.co.uk/confs.htm)**
The site contains a listing of conferences organised by the RCN in the UK and Europe.

### Royal College of Nursing UK
### (http://www.rcn.org.uk)

The RCN is the world's largest professional union for registered nurses, midwives and health visitors. The site provides information about the organisation and a service for members who require professional, legal and education advice.

### Royal Windsor Society for Nursing Research ('For Your Information')
### (http://www.windsor.igs.net/~nhodgins)

The site is a useful new resource designed to promote nursing research at a global level. It includes online workshops, a nursing journals database and newsgroup. There is also a listing of professional services and opportunities and recent publications. There are plans to include an online workshop on database design/software choice as well as a basic nursing research study website design.

### UK Central Council (UKCC)
### (http:www.healthworks.co.uk/hw/orgs/UKCC.html)

The site contains information on the organisation, structure, funding and membership of the UKCC plus contact details.

### Welsh National Board for Nursing, Midwifery and Health Visiting
### (http://www.wnb.org.uk)

The site provides information relevant to nurses, midwives and health visitors working in Wales and also those wishing to enter the profession.

### Worldwide Nurse
### (http://www.wwnurse.com)

This is a valuable site with an extensive compilation of links to online nursing sites and journals, colleges and universities, lists of employment vacancies and nursing humour.

(Reproduced, with alterations, with kind permission from Baillière's Nurses' Dictionary 23e, Weller (ed), 2000, Baillière Tindall).

# Index